D0599395

A WOMAN'S GUIDE TO

# Tantra Yoga

# A WOMAN'S GUIDE TO
# *Tantra Yoga*

Vimala McClure

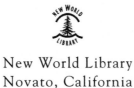

New World Library
Novato, California

New World Library
14 Pamaron Way
Novato, CA 94949

© 1997 Vimala McClure

Cover illustration by Pam Rossi
Cover and text design by Aaron Kenedi
Illustrations by Michael B. McClure

All rights reserved. This book may not be
reproduced in whole or in part, or transmitted in any form,
or by any means electronic, mechanical, photocopying,
recording, or other, without written permission from the
publisher, except by a reviewer who may quote
brief passages in a review.

**Library of Congress Cataloging-in-Publication Data**

McClure, Vimala Schneider, 1952 —
(Some still want the moon)
A woman's guide to tantra yoga / Vimala McClure.
p.  cm.
Originally published: Some still want the moon. Willow Springs, MO :
Nucleus Publications, 1989
ISBN 1-57731-017-9 (pbk. : alk. paper)
1. Yoga. 2. Tantrism. 3. Women — Conduct of life. I. Title.

[b132.Y6M373  1997]                                              96-54836
291.4'36—dc21                                                        CIP

First printing, May 1997
Printed in Canada on acid-free paper
ISBN 1-57731-017-9
Distributed to the trade by Publishers Group West
10  9  8  7  6  5  4  3  2  1

Dedicated to P. R. Sarkar

# Acknowledgments

The author wishes to thank Michael McClure, Joni Zweig, Tom Barefoot, Christina Davis, and Barbara Parham for their help and support.

# Contents

Contents

# An Invitation

In 1971, I was nineteen years old. After a tumultuous adolescence I was searching for some positive direction for my life. A creek ran by the small house where I lived and I sat by it every day that summer, trying to unravel the truth about life and my place in it. I began reading books about yoga, which led me to an interest in adopting a vegetarian diet. One day in the health food store I saw a notice for a free yoga class. I took the class and was so impressed by the instructor and by the changes that a simple daily routine of yoga and meditation brought into my life that I continued to study and practice. Eventually I began to teach, and my curiosity led me to India, where I met my spiritual teacher and transformed my life through study of the teachings of the vast body of work called Tantra Yoga, and through service to the poor.

Many years and many changes have occurred in my life since then, but one constant is my daily practice. Tantric meditation has provided me with a spiritual base upon which I have built the rest of my life. It is a daily alchemy, turning the dross of my mind's wanderings into the golden treasure of spiritual realization. I cannot imagine my life without this treasure. I have not had an easy life, nor have I always understood the meaning of its trials, but my meditation has always brought me into focus, provided me with strength to prevail over pain and loss, and inspired me to continue to find my way to health and positivity. It has nurtured my desire to contribute whatever I can to the betterment of my world, and helped me to find creative ways to do so. The intuitive capabilities I have developed and the love I feel for people (which allows me to communicate well with parents and babies with whom I often work as an educator and counselor) are a direct result of my daily spiritual work.

A book like this one introduced me to Tantra Yoga, its underlying philosophy, and the benefits of meditation. This book explores a wide range of areas, sometimes with the perspective of Western science, sometimes with teachings from the East. I go into depth with a variety of things — and not all of them may interest you at this stage of your life. That's fine — just skip over what doesn't grab your attention at the moment, and read and reflect on what does.

I wrote this book with a desire to provide other women with an invitation. The words certainly apply to men as well: No one can walk your spiritual path for you; each step must be taken consciously, by you alone. No guru, guide, or channel can do the inner work that is necessary to develop your higher capabilities and bring you to the realization that answers your deepest questions. Make yourself very still, and listen quietly with openness. You will be led to what you need at every point along the way.

# What Is Tantra Yoga?

Tantra is the oldest Eastern tradition of spiritual philosophy and practice, having originated more than 7,000 years ago in India. From its origin to the present day, it is a revolutionary approach to human evolution. The word *Tantra* means liberation through mental expansion, and the word *yoga* means union, in this case the unity of the self and all creation with the source of all being. The basic tenet of Tantra is that all of life is food for spiritual development, from the most mundane tasks of everyday living to the deepest meditation. Tantra teaches us to embrace life, to strive to see the Creator in everything within and around us. The practices, including concentration, meditation, yoga postures, relaxation, visualization, nourishing food, community involvement, service, and right conduct, are all designed to help us experience body, mind, spirit, joy, peace, suffering, and pain as changing aspects of one indivisible Being.

You may have heard Tantra referred to as the "yoga of sex." While sexuality is a part of Tantra because it is a part of life, it is not the core of Tantric philosophy or practice. In Chapter Seven, we will examine this issue more closely, clarifying the underlying tradition that led to this misinterpretation of Tantra's focus and meaning. Practitioners of Tantra often refer to it as the "yoga of everything." Unlike many religious philosophies that separate the spiritual from the mundane by rejecting that which is not overtly spiritual, Tantra teaches us that in order to realize our oneness with the Supreme Being we must accept, not reject. We must embrace life in all of its struggle and pain, and through this profound acceptance we will find peace and experience freedom from the bondage of self-imposed limitation.

# Chapter One
## Your Perfect Nature

*Some people, no matter what you give them, still want the moon.*
— Denise Levertov, *Adam's Complaint*

### CONSCIOUSNESS

Gaze, for a while, at the vast expanse of the ocean. Its surface is turbulent, waves crashing, spewing millions of water droplets into the air. But as you dive deeper, the turbulence subsides; at its depths is silence and peace. Ordinarily you may experience only the surface of your mind's potential — the crashing waves of emotion, millions of thoughts like tiny drops of water flying in every direction. Meditation helps you dive deeply into your mind, and in the process, uncover hidden treasures.

As you discover the deeper aspects of your mind, you become better able to control your thoughts, your actions, and your reactions to the external world. "Who am I?" "Where did I come from?" and "Why am I here?" are questions whose answers are revealed as your feeling of individual existence merges with infinite awareness.

In another way, your mind is like the ocean reflecting the image of the moon. It is possible to see the reflection of the moon on the water only when the water is calm, not when the waves are turbulent. Similarly, pure consciousness is only revealed when your mind is calm and still, when the agitated waves of thought and desire cease.

The old materialistic concepts about the origin and composition of mind and matter are dissolving as we learn that matter is nothing but bottled-up energy, a pattern of waves in endless motion. Everything, from matter to thought, is made up of these waves. Physicists are beginning to recognize that intelligence is at the source of all creation. Physicist Lincoln Barnett was perhaps speaking of the connection between matter and spirit when he said, "In the evolution of scientific thought one fact has become impressively clear: there is no mystery of the physical world which does not point to a mystery beyond itself." Through the science of intuition, or the practice of meditation, you explore these mysteries, discovering the subtle substance from which the universe evolves, which we call infinite consciousness, or *Brahma*.

## YOUR PERFECT NATURE

There is a hunger for limitless freedom and happiness within every person. We seek freedom from the bondage of time, place, and person. We want to surmount time, replacing walking with supersonic travel; we try to expand our spatial boundaries with instantaneous communication and transport systems, stretching even into outer space. We attempt to surpass our personal limitations with dramas, masks, stories, personal love (trying to merge with another) and with endless attempts to create the "new me." All these attempts lead to exploration, invention, and efforts at social, political, economic, and sexual freedom. But the only absolute freedom is to go beyond material progress and reach for expanded consciousness.

This reaching, this search for something greater, is our innate nature, our *dharma*. Everything in the universe has its nature. Dharma is that which maintains the structural integrity of something, without which that entity could not exist. The innate nature of fire is its capacity to burn. The nature of most of the animal kingdom is to eat, drink, procreate, and sleep; various species have their species-specific dharma, such as the honey-making nature of bees.

The most significant quality that sets human beings apart from animals has to do with the evolution of our minds; we can call it our "perfect nature." We, too, have the animal instincts for self-preservation, but we also have a longing for the Great. It is that part of you that remains unsatisfied with appeasing the animal instincts, that propels you toward fulfillment — the search for infinite happiness. But unending happiness and self-actualization can never be yours by simply fulfilling your desires with material things or intellectual ideas, which are finite. Even personal relationships are temporary; your family and dearest friends will one day pass away. The only way the desire for infinite happiness can be fulfilled is by establishing yourself in the infinite, by merging your consciousness with all-knowing supreme consciousness. Whether you consciously know it or not, this is your goal. This is where your perfect nature is taking you.

## THE FOUR PARTS OF YOUR PERFECT NATURE

According to the ancient teachings of Tantra, there are four components of your perfect nature: expansion of mind, vibrational flow, selfless service, and consciousness. Meditation is the practical means whereby your perfect nature can be realized. Meditation helps you, step by step, through specific practices, to achieve that realization.

First you learn the practice of mental expansion (called *vistara* in Sanskrit). As you go about your day-to-day activities the mind is absorbed in countless objects and sense impressions. No matter how hard you try, you will find it impossible to stop this natural flow of your mind. It is always jumping from one thing to another, often in such a manner as to work itself into a frenzy, creating both physical and mental stress. The Indian saint Ramakrishna once characterized the mind as "a mad monkey stung by a scorpion." The mind must always have an object; you can use this natural tendency and give it an "infinite object" on which to focus.

The ego, or the part of the mind that can say, "I exist," is always focused on the external world. The consciousness — the part of you that can say, "I know I exist" — witnesses the ego's activity. When you meditate, you reverse the outward-going process, training your mind to focus instead on the infinite, beyond form or thought. The ego makes you feel as if you are a separate individual entity. It must have a finite object or thought with which to be involved in order to maintain its existence. Given infinite consciousness as its object, the individual sense of "I" merges with the infinite "I." It is unable to contain this feeling of infinite awareness within the limited scope of its existence. What evolves from this practice is a state of absolute peace, which is beyond description because it is beyond the busy workings of the mind.

The outward expression of mental expansion is the realization of the oneness of all creation. This universal outlook prevents you from encouraging any division in humanity. You are inspired from within to work for the unity and elevation of all and to remove the barriers that separate living beings from one another. Expansion of mind lends compassion to your outlook and enables you to accept the problems of the world as your own.

The second aspect of your perfect nature can be called "vibrational flow" (called *rasa* in Sanskrit). This sounds a little esoteric. What does it mean? We know from physics, as well as from Eastern teachings, that everything in the universe is composed of vibration.

According to Tantra, your mind, as well as the physical universe, is made of the thought waves of infinite consciousness. Nothing is truly external. In each being, the combination of all its wavelengths — physical, mental, emotional — is its individual vibration. Each of us, because of our previous experiences, our environment, our desires, and stage of development, has an entirely different vibrational expression than any other being. But infinite consciousness is beyond all of our individual tendencies. Infinite consciousness is the combination of every vibration in the universe; its vibrational flow is the flow of the entire cosmos.

Another important component of meditation comes into play here: "living meditation," the practice of merging your individual rhythmic vibration with that of the infinite, while trying to keep your mind immersed in that flow at all times. You come to realize that your individual flow is that of the Supreme, and so all of your actions are in harmony with it.

Happiness, attraction, or congeniality results when the vibrational expression of one being is harmonious with that of another. Conversely, irritation, stress, even hatred results when those same vibrational rhythms oppose or clash with one another. You've probably experienced a sense of being "in tune" with someone ("I liked you from the moment I met you") — or the opposite ("The minute I saw him, I knew we wouldn't get along"). When you are able to bring your individual vibrational rhythms into harmony with infinite consciousness, an inner calm and happiness ensues that is not affected by the finite world. Your understanding of others increases. You are in harmony with the creator of all vibrational expressions, and you are able to adjust your own expressions accordingly. Thus, you are no longer tossed about by attraction and repulsion, but empathy, understanding, and deep love for all creation gives you a pleasure much finer than you have ever experienced.

The third part of your perfect nature is selfless service (called *seva* in Sanskrit). Service is giving fully of yourself without expectation of reward. It is the result of mental expansion and vibrational flow. The person who meditates regularly eventually gains the expansion of mind to perceive consciousness in all creation. She also gains the harmonious relationship with the universe that enables her to work selflessly for its evolution and transformation.

Service and meditation are like two lovers who are never happily separated. It is impossible to progress in meditation without developing the impulse to care for others; the universal love that grows as a result of the mind's expansion compels us to serve. Service is an extension of meditation. The thought, "I am an expression of infinite consciousness, serving the infinite in you" helps to uplift the mind and prepare it for meditation. When you serve, your thought is that "infinite consciousness has manifested before me in this form in order to give me a chance to serve." In this way the limited ego is kept in perspective, the mind is immersed in the thought of oneness, progress in meditation is assured, and your service ensures the progress of your fellow beings.

The fourth and final aspect of your perfect nature is actually the goal — infinite consciousness (*parama purusa*). It is your very essence. It is perfection.

Although every living being, every atom, cell, and subatomic particle, every rock, every plant, everything in the universe is in essence that consciousness, we humans have the unique capacity to know our divinity, to realize our perfection in the spiritual realm. This faculty also gives us a responsibility to the world in which we live: to develop ourselves to fulfill our great potential.

This sense of oneness with the infinite is more than mood-making. Fritjof Capra writes, in *The Tao of Physics*, "The basic oneness of the universe is not only the central characteristic of the mystical experience, but is also one of the most important revelations of modern physics." Many physicists and others who study the origins of the universe are coming to the conclusion that oneness is the natural state from which everything arises.

## ATTITUDE

Meditation is not a magic cure-all that can be taken in doses to work overnight. Your approach is definitely an important factor in your self-realization. Although there is no failure in meditation, your attitude can make the difference between ease and difficulty. Cultivating the right frame of mind is very helpful if you are serious about continuing your practice, because it supplies the internal inspiration and enthusiasm that will fuel your meditation and color your thoughts and actions throughout each day.

The essence of Tantra Yoga is the joyous affirmation that "there is nothing that is not divine." Instead of proclaiming, like many traditional philosophies, "God is not this, God is not that," the Tantric affirms, "All is God; I am God." By recognizing that all forms in the universe are manifestations of the same consciousness, your attitude becomes positive and dynamic. You see the universe as the arena for spiritual endeavor. Perceived and utilized properly, it

*I*n the progress toward truth, let us notice that each step is from particles to waves, or from material to mental; the final picture consists wholly of waves, and its ingredients are wholly mental constructs. It seems more and more likely that reality is better described as mental than material.

— Physicist James Jeans

reveals, not veils, God. Rather than concentrating on admonitions of "don't be this way, don't do that," you concentrate on the positive, using all your physical, mental, and spiritual potential as part of your path. Meditation is not a process of elimination, but of inclusion, expanding your awareness of that consciousness infinitely.

## DISCRIMINATION AND NONATTACHMENT

You might think that to such a person, discrimination and nonattachment would be negative concepts. But understood properly these two functions of the higher mind are integral to the positive approach of Tantra Yoga.

Discrimination is knowing what is lasting and what is not, being able to perceive the eternal consciousness within the passing show of the material world, and knowing that attachment to finite objects ultimately can only bring pain and suffering. In this age, it is increasingly easy for us to remain aloof from suffering and death. Because we are not faced with it every day, we become oblivious to our connection with it. We fail to realize that one day we too must die — we too must suffer the pain of loss. The impersonal way in which we are exposed to pain and death, via movies and television, only serves to further separate us from its reality and to desensitize us to the suffering of others.

When faced with the shock of loss, we long for some kind of eternal base for our lives — for the knowledge that will enable us to understand these events and thus cope with our fear and loneliness. Many people turn to religion, but turn away again after their crisis has passed and their mental stability has been restored. This is because often religion can offer only a temporary solace that is no real base in itself. Religions that require faith that is not firmly rooted in personal experience or knowledge, that do not give specific practices by which that knowledge is acquired, often fail to offer the continuing growth and the real answers that the rational individual seeks.

Meditation is a practical connecting link to the eternal base. Rather than acting as a crutch in times of distress, it is a tool with which you can find real answers from within. The realization achieved through meditation is not faith or belief, but knowledge, and as scientists, psychologists, and philosophers have shown us, fear and all of its accompanying anxiety can only be banished by knowledge. The realization attained through meditation enlightens religious beliefs, enabling you to understand the deeper meaning of your chosen religious teachings and apply them to your life.

When that connecting link is established through meditation and you gain some personal experience of your goal, you will begin to gain a sense of discrimination — the ability to place finite events and objects in their proper perspective with the infinite from which they have all evolved.

As it reveals the subtler aspects of your mind, meditation brings you to this fine sense of discrimination, which in turn leads to nonattachment. According to some philosophies, nonattachment means avoidance of the things of the world. Thus some spiritual seekers have mortified themselves to renounce the pleasure and pain of the body; have tried to create aversions in their minds to the natural instincts of eating, sleeping, and sexuality; and have escaped from society to live in jungles or caves far from the "temptations" of worldly life.

Volumes of psychiatric research have shown us that repression is never successful. Such methods of dealing with attachment merely create more obstacles for the practitioner, because they require the mind to be absorbed in negative thoughts rather than in truth. If you adopt such measures you will ultimately turn away from your goal; repression forces your mind to be more deeply entrenched in those things from which you are trying to escape. Although solitude may remove you from the immediate agitations of the world, it does not remove those agitations from the mind, which is their source.

Meditation can reveal truth and calm the agitations of the mind, and it can be practiced anywhere. True detachment is never a negative approach; rather it is a positive attitude of love for the goal, seeing universal consciousness in all forms, and attaching the mind to that infinite essence rather than the finite form in which it appears.

Negative interpretations of discrimination and nonattachment developed through the ages as a result of priest-classes controlling spiritual practice and knowledge. It was expedient for them to retain their power and prestige by preventing ordinary family people from practicing meditation, especially women, who historically have been most "attached" because of their guardianship of home and children. Even today many people avoid meditation because they associate it with solitary asceticism and detachment.

Discrimination also means understanding that pleasure is not the goal of our existence. You can, rather, identify with the broader context within which both pleasure and pain exist as polar expressions. Your attitude is one of dynamic simplicity. You strive without ambition, neither avoiding pain nor seeking pleasure but accepting yourself as you are, letting the process of meditation unfold all of your potentialities naturally within you. Meditation helps you to live your life in balance, and a balanced mind gains deeper realization in meditation.

## MOTIVATION

When the realization of oneness develops within, a feeling of attraction for the goal intensifies. As you begin to understand yourself and the universe, as your perfect nature unfolds, you realize that a magnetic attraction to infinite consciousness or truth is the force that has guided you from the beginning of your life. This same force is the essential energy of the universe, which keeps everything moving in perfect balance. This realization will awaken in you a special kind of love.

Until now, you have been pulled along the path of progress purely by the force of evolution. At a certain point, though, you are bound to discover that the force that is pulling you is infinite consciousness, your innermost being. This discovery is one of great joy, and you begin to use more of your own conscious energy to move toward your goal. It is as if you have been lost in a forest, finding your way home only by vague feelings, memories, and landmarks along the way. You wander slowly, carefully, sometimes taking wrong turns, stumbling, confused. But when in the distance the light of home can be seen, you cry out joyfully and run straight for that light, all doubts gone, confusion and loneliness replaced by joyful anticipation and relief. No longer is every fallen log an obstacle, every dark corner a menace, every divergent path a temptation. You return home with speed and confidence. The awakening of devotion — intense love for the higher self — in the heart of the spiritual seeker is such an experience. With it a new relationship develops between you and your spiritual goal that changes the very quality of your meditative practice.

Psychologist Abraham Maslow described these two stages of motivation as "deficiency" motivation and "growth" or "being" motivation, and the two different kinds of love they produce as "deficiency-love" and "being-love."

Deficiency-motivated living is based on needs that must be met from without and by others — the need for security, respect, and acceptance. It is an attitude of defending and preserving oneself, of fending off attack rather than reaching out for fulfillment. Deficiency love (called *kama* in yoga terminology) is based on the need of the limited ego; it can be grasping, fearful, insecure. It is an emptiness that must be filled.

Growth — or being-motivation is something different; however, it is not contradictory. One passes into the other as childhood passes into maturity. The growth-motivated individual has seen the light of home and no longer feels that previous emptiness. Secure and self-directed, with growth-motivation you are able to fully give of yourself because you are no longer motivated by fear. This change does not, however, mean you are exempt from conflict or unhappiness. As a growth-motivated person, you are better able to deal with conflict through meditation and self-searching. Thus, from this perspective, you are better able to see problems clearly and be open to accepting help, when necessary, from outside sources. Being-love, or *prema* is fearless. You love the essence, the being, rather than its changing physical attributes or its capacity to fill the ego's needs. It is open and selfless, and ultimately, beyond the limitations of the emotions or the physical body.

The infinite consciousness within you seeks expression. When you begin to live your life in a way that allows your higher nature to unfold, door after door will open to you. Others begin to seek you out because of your harmonizing energies. You live, work, and play from a center of focused attention that not only allows you to experience limitless energy and tranquility but draws into your world only the best for you.

## ARE YOU BOUND BY FATE?

Throw a rock into a pool of still, clear water. What happens? The water reacts. It changes shape, emanating rings of waves that are strongest at the point of contact. The reflection of the moon above is broken up into a thousand moving pieces, made unrecognizable.

The mind is always in a state of motion, experiencing the reactions of previous thoughts and actions, like rocks thrown incessantly into the peaceful stillness of a pool. Meditation helps you to put down the rock, let the waters settle, and peer in to see the beautiful reflection of your perfect nature. When you experience this oneness with infinite consciousness, you begin to free yourself from the shackles of so-called fate.

Throughout the ages, people have sought to explain the seemingly random occurrences in their lives. Some religions teach that God (often perceived as a stern, manlike figure in the sky) rewards the virtuous and punishes those who sin. These philosophies must undergo tremendous contortions of logic to withstand the questions of rational people. Hindu "fatalists" assert that every action has its consequences and the sufferings of this life have their prologue in previous incarnations. But because of the limitations of religious dogma, these ideas spawned the caste system in India, whereby millions of people have suffered, kept ignorant and poor by the dictum that it was their fate, decreed by the gods. Better luck next life! Newton's famous assertion that for every action there is an opposite reaction is a basic physical law that applies on the level of mind as well. The mind's balance is constantly disturbed by thoughts, actions, impressions. It seeks to regain its original state and strives with force to correct imbalances.

Every thought or action reaps its reaction. Nothing is lost. The universe,

Do you love your son? That is perfectly correct. But on the son's death you will have great pain. Isn't that also correct? The son is a finite entity. He cannot live until eternity. He will depart and leave you. But if you treat your son as the expression of God in the form of your son, then there will never be any fear of losing him because God can never be lost. It is present around you in all directions. In that state of mind you will be able to give proper treatment to whatever finite being you come in contact with.

— P. R. Sarkar

according to the theory of relativity, is curved in on itself. If you could throw an object into space with enough force, it would traverse the universe and come round again to hit you in the back of the head. In the same way, every vibration emanating from you — whether thought, word, or action — will return, with force, to affect your life for good or ill. These potential reactions, called *samskaras*, are the results of thoughts and actions. They remain stored in the mind until mature and are then experienced as "the forces of blind fate." They have their own energy, their own momentum. According to Tantric teachings, this momentum — more accurately called "reactive momenta" — can only mature when the mind is dissociated from its incessant concern with the physical body, as in unconsciousness or death. In the state after death, when the mind is dissociated from the body, momenta from the previous life mature, and when the soul incarnates again in a suitable physical body, those reactions are experienced and new ones are created. Thus the wheel of birth and death turns ceaselessly.

In meditation you momentarily dissociate yourself from concern with the physical body, not in simulation of death, but by identifying with the eternal source of all life. This is another opportunity for reactive momenta to mature. But within your practice lies the key that will stop the relentless turning of the wheel. Each time you meditate, some of the reactive momenta mature. Returning to your everyday life, you experience these reactions, reaping what you have sown in this and previous lives. This is why sometimes, especially in the beginning, the new practitioner faces a period of difficulties and obstacles. She undergoes more reactions than the ordinary person. But this phase passes, leaving the meditator freer than before; fewer and fewer potential reactions are created as her meditation gains strength and concentration.

The more you meditate, the more you attain equilibrium in every sphere of your life. You begin to perceive the same infinite consciousness pervading all, and thus your mind isn't disturbed by any situation. With no disturbance, there is no need to correct the disturbance, no reaction. Meditation ripens the old reactive momenta and enables you to stop creating new ones. By experiencing your old reactions without attachment, you let them go. Eventually all of your old reactions are exhausted and no new ones appear to be experienced. Your mind has achieved a state of peace, and the body is no longer needed as a vehicle for the expression of reactive momenta. At the end of a practitioner's life, her reactions are finished, and, upon leaving her earthly body, her mind merges into infinite consciousness.

## THE THREE TYPES OF REACTIONS

There are three types of reactions in potentiality: inborn, acquired, and imposed. The inborn reactions are those we have acquired in previous lives. A child prodigy is one who probably developed a great degree of proficiency in her past life.

Acquired reactions are those you create of your own will, through action independent of your inborn reactive momenta. A young woman grows up in a family of chefs and has culinary talent from an early age. However, she may acquire momentum to earn her degree in physics and spend her life studying quark symmetries.

Imposed reactions are the impressions created upon your mind by the world in which you live. You acquire these as you are influenced by world conditions, family, responsibility, and education. The young woman in the previous example will always be a good cook because of the momentum imposed by her chef parents.

Peer groups can impose reactive momenta, as can teachers and elders. Thus education and environment are very important to the growing child. The combination of inborn momenta — heredity, through genetic material, is an expression of these — and those that are acquired and imposed all propel a child into her future as an adult. Acquired and imposed reactions have a tremendous effect on how the inborn reactions are expressed. It is crucial that every child have the food, clothing, shelter, education, and medical attention she needs; this is one reason we strive to serve those less fortunate than ourselves. Fate has not decreed the suffering of the poor, the homeless, or hungry. These reactive momenta are forced upon people by their environment and by the lack of opportunities to acquire the momentum for physical, mental, and spiritual well-being.

Children are particularly vulnerable to the imposition of reactive momenta; they are easily affected by constant contact with external forces. For example, a child may come into the world with the momentum for a tremendous amount of physical activity. Her environment, however, will have an impact upon how that activity manifests. She could be a great athlete, or she might be a violent criminal.

As adults we have acquired a certain amount of defensive psychological armor against others' impositions on us. But without the strength and clarity of mind afforded by daily meditation we are still vulnerable to imposition by stronger minds than our own. During Hitler's reign, a few concentrated minds imposed the most ghastly samskaras on millions of people.

On a smaller scale, you may find yourself mesmerized every day, often unknowingly influenced by values subliminally imposed upon you through advertising, political double-talk, music, and media hype. Meditation helps you gain the clarity to see through the hype and to acquire the tools to defuse its impact in your life and the lives of your children. It inspires you to create uplifting environments and to seek the most expansive expressions in art, music, and literature for yourself and for all of humanity.

Reactive momenta differentiates one person from another. We are all essentially the same consciousness; the course our lives take is a combination of our free will here and now (momenta we acquire in this life) and what we have chosen in the past. Our desires and prayers can often create reactions that we, with our limited view, cannot perceive in advance, as we earnestly pray for our dreams to come true. A friend of mine once wanted a television. She had a strong mind, having practiced meditation and yoga for several years. Soon after this desire came into her mind, a neighbor knocked on her door.

"My parents are moving today," the neighbor said, "and they have a television they don't need any more. I thought maybe you'd like to have it." "Sure!" said my friend, amazed at how quickly her desire had manifested. They brought the television into the living room and set it down. My friend stared at it, horrified. It was a huge, ugly, old-fashioned television, and it was pink. And when she turned it on, nothing happened — it didn't work! She kept that pink television for a long time, to remind herself to always be aware of how she used her mind.

Our reactive momenta take us from one lifetime to the next, determining the wavelength of our earthly body (and thus its characteristics, through the genes) as well as the family, environment, and social structure into which we are born. Like water poured into different cups, consciousness takes the shape of you or me. When the cups are emptied, the water merges, and all is One.

## A NOTE ON REINCARNATION

It is not necessary to believe in reincarnation in order to meditate and to lead a spiritual life. An abundance of evidence points to its validity; however, defining the philosophical structure on which it is based is another book and cannot be my intention here. Do your own research, setting aside acquired prejudices in a sincere effort to know the truth. There is no need to commit yourself to a firm belief. Your meditation will eventually reveal to you the truth of all existence.

Your spiritual life does not depend on belief but on practice. Whether you believe in one life or ten billion, your practice of meditation will still have wonderful results — some you will experience almost immediately, and some will gradually unfold over time.

Recommended Reading:

*The Tao of Physics* by Fritjof Capra

*Einstein's Space and Van Gogh's Sky: Physical Reality and Beyond* by Lawrence LeShan and Henry Margeneau

*Reincarnation: a New Horizon in Science, Religion, and Society* by Sylvia Cranston and Carey Williams

*Up from Eden* by Ken Wilbur

# Chapter Two
# The Circle of Love

*We all come from God, and unto God do we return, like a stream flowing back to the ocean, like a ray of light returning to the sun.* — Quaker hymn

## THE CREATION OF THE UNIVERSE

There is a consciousness in the grass and trees, a consciousness that animates the tiny amoeba, that manifests in the amazing animal kingdom and in the wondrous richness of human life. This consciousness permeates all creation, from the deepest recesses of our earth to the farthest unknown galaxy. It controls the movement of the stars and it blossoms in the tiniest flower. It creates, it maintains, and it destroys, and yet it is beyond even these. We can call it *Brahma*, the Supreme. In the ancient science of Tantra, the creation of the universe is a cycle, called *Brahmachakra* — the "circle of the Supreme."

There are two parts of the cycle of creation: the "extroversal" phase of expansion, when pure consciousness manifests into matter and mind, and the "introversal" phase, when that consciousness slowly returns to its pure state. Along the way there are temporary reversals, but the essential evolution is from infinite consciousness into static matter and back to consciousness again.

When you begin to understand this cycle, you can begin to perceive the roots of all scientific and religious thought. Researchers, physicists, philosophers, and religious teachers through the ages have discovered pieces of the puzzle of creation and have labeled them in many ways, making it look as if there are many distinctly different theories of creation. But if you study carefully, you will begin to see that the pieces of the puzzle fit together. Many creation stories are simply the attempts of early teachers to translate subtle ideas into symbols that people of their day could understand.

Modern thinkers are beginning to piece together more of the creation and evolution theories, and what is emerging looks very much like yoga philosophy. Ken Wilbur, author of such groundbreaking books as *The Spectrum of Consciousness* and *Up from Eden,* maintains that the force of evolution is the drive toward spirit. "The creation did not take place all at once at some time in the distant past," he says. "Creation is occurring now as evolution — ceaselessly novel, ceaselessly driving toward higher and higher unities in search of the absolute Unity, or spirit itself. And that, I believe, is the only way to bring science and religion together." According to Tantra this ultimate unity is Brahma, and every being, every atom in the universe is moving toward realization of that supreme state.

Try to picture the infinite cycle of creation in your imagination. Go way back, before the beginning, before matter, before mind . . . oops! You've hit a snag already. How can you, with the mind, perceive that which is beyond the mind? The point between manifest and unmanifest consciousness is the "beginning" of the creation of the universe — a point not in time but beyond it. Only through deep meditation can you perceive this initial point, and when you do, you merge in it and you are unable to communicate that state in words. A knotty problem!

Speaking of knotty problems, I want to share with you a dilemma I encountered while writing this chapter. Tantric cosmology is fascinating and complex. It combines quantum physics, intuitive insight, and religious metaphor. Much of it is not yet understood in scientific terms. I have tried to get it into simple language and to eliminate as many Sanskrit words as possible, but, quite frankly, it's still rough going. I considered placing it at the end of the book, but these concepts are the foundation upon which the practices of yoga and meditation are built. Understanding the cycle of creation is, in my view, very helpful — though not essential — in motivating you to do meditation and yoga practices every day. It provides a context for the conduct of everyday life.

So, it's up to you: You can either read on from here, or skip over this chapter and read the rest of the book, referring back to this one when you need the information.

## What Is Supreme Consciousness Made Of?

Brahma is composed of cosmic consciousness, called *Shiva,* and cosmic energy, called *Shakti,* and it exists in two states. Like flowers and their fragrance or fire and its burning, Shiva and Shakti are inseparable. Understanding this oneness is essential. Religion often divorces Shiva from Shakti, saying that God and creation are different and separate. But both Tantric science and modern physics contend that consciousness is one, whether manifest or unmanifest.

In the very beginning Brahma is so pure that it has no sense of existence. It is beyond anything we can imagine. Shakti, the latent creative force, is composed of three tendencies or forces. The *sentient tendency* imparts the sense of existence and also the feelings of happiness and relief. It awakens the desire to seek liberation from bondage. It is the force of life, of luster and beauty. The *mutative tendency* is the sense of action, of growth; it activates the "I." The *static tendency* is that which gives the results of action, which binds action to reaction. It is the force of stagnation and death.

These transforming qualities are apparent in every object of the created universe. One of these is always dominant, as the play of forces moves from one to the other. The life force of the mutative tendency is what dominates as a flower blossoms in the spring. As long as the mutative tendency prevails, the sentient tendency glows from within. But when the force of the mutative tendency is spent, the static tendency predominates, and the luster of the sentient tendency fades; the flower wilts and dies.

## THE CREATION OF COSMIC MIND

Imagine Shiva, or pure consciousness, to be like the ocean, and Shakti, or creative energy, like the climate. When the climate is stable, or congruent with the ocean, the water flows freely, uninhibited. This is the state before the beginning — the state of absolute peace. The transforming principles of Shakti flow in Shiva without obstruction. But at some point the climatic conditions change and freeze a part of this ocean. The transforming factors gradually form a matrix, and the forces begin to play. The sentient tendency converts to mutative, the mutative to static, the static to mutative and, eventually, back to sentient again, thus creating a whirlpool of balanced but interacting forces. This interaction becomes a struggle for dominance, and, because it is the most powerful of the three, the sentient force prevails.

At this subtle point, Shakti begins to transform Shiva with its forces, and pure consciousness manifests in its first stage: cosmic mind. There begins to emerge in this ocean of consciousness the feeling of existence: "I am." It is only after this self-awareness occurs that creation can begin; the sense of existence is necessary for action. This sense of "I am" has come about as a result of the subtlest transforming factor, the sentient tendency, exerting the first influence upon consciousness.

Now that the "I am" exists, Shakti's energy continues to transform even further with the mutative tendency. The water of our imaginary ocean has gone from free-flowing to dense, and now it is ... slush! The influence of the mutative tendency enables cosmic mind to act. "I am" becomes "I do." Now the mutative tendency has full sway over consciousness; the final transforming force takes over. The pressure of the static tendency objectifies a portion of cosmic mind in order to act. This objectified portion is mind-stuff (*ectoplasm*). Cosmic mind-stuff is the iceberg in the ocean. The subtlest consciousness is now ready to be transformed into dense material forms.

The combination of the sense of "I am," the sense of "I do," and the cosmic ectoplasm is called cosmic mind, and it is through the thought waves of the cosmic mind that the innumerable forms of the created universe come into existence. But the entire creation doesn't just burst forth from the "imagination" of Brahma. It is a natural, creative process, and like all creative endeavors, the stage must be set; the requisite conditions must be created first.

Before a baby is born, all of the right conditions must exist in its mother's womb: the right temperature, the right time in the mother's cycle, even the pull of the moon can affect the conception, growth, and birth of a child. If conditions are favorable, microscopic cells divide and become an embryo, which in turn unfolds, in a perfectly designed sequence, all of the elements necessary for the development of a human being. So, too, in the creation of the universe, the subtlest factors must first exist before the denser forms, which we can perceive, can come into being. These are the five fundamental factors, the basic building-blocks of the manifest universe.

## THE BUILDING BLOCKS OF THE UNIVERSE

As the influence of Shakti's static principle transforms consciousness more and more, a portion of cosmic mind densifies and becomes the etheric factor or what we term "space." Space is the stuff in which the universe exists; it is the subtlest substance. It has the capacity to carry the subtlest quality, that of sound — even though, in pure space, it is not yet audible.

The static tendency continues exerting more and more influence within a portion of space and transforms it into the next denser factor: air. The aerial factor can carry the vibrational essences of both sound and touch. Air gives sound the ability to touch the ear; thus, sound becomes audible at this stage. Atoms of hydrogen come into being, and the pressure of the static force draws them together, forming hydrogen clouds. The force of gravity causes the clouds to condense, which drives the atoms closer together, causing friction and heat. This is the first expression of the next denser factor: luminosity.

The luminous factor carries the vibrational qualities of sound, touch, and sight. Thus light comes into being, and stars are born. At this stage the increasing heat and pressure at the center of a star fuses the hydrogen nuclei together to make helium. Later heavier atoms are fused and each of the elements is created. The space between atoms and molecules continues to decrease, eventually condensing the luminous factor into liquid plasma.

The liquid factor carries the sensory qualities of sound, touch, sight, and taste. Further pressure from the static tendency solidifies the liquid factor, and the solid factor — carrying the vibration of smell as well — comes into being. At this point all the factors coexist simultaneously in the universe. The degree and combinations of these five factors determines the makeup of all material substances and how the next act in the drama of creation evolves.

## THE PRESSURE THAT CREATES LIFE

To this point, the creative process has been *extroversal* (meaning "the whole moving outward") — movement from subtle to dense. Inanimate matter is the densest form of consciousness. Shakti's static force can transform no further, and its hold must begin to loosen. The *introversal* phase of creation (meaning "the whole moving inward") begins as matter finds its way back to pure consciousness again.

The static tendency exerts so much pressure on the solid factor that a tension of forces is created. The center-seeking force of static Shakti clashes with the force of expansion, which is directed from the center outward. These two forces vie for dominance, and a critical climax in the cycle of creation occurs. If the force of expansion becomes dominant, the structure can no longer maintain the delicate balance, and it dissociates into billions of particles.

On the other hand, if there is an imbalance of the five factors within the structure, the object contracts more and more, the tension in the solid factor becomes very great, and an explosion occurs. At this point the densest factor is converted back into subtler factors to "try again." This means, of course, that no factors are lost. The eventual death of the universe, therefore, is impossible. Furthermore, cosmic mind is never imperiled by the explosions in the dense factor; the particles return to their respective factors. Cosmic mind-stuff remains unaffected, and creation continues endlessly.

The alternative course is that which, when it occurs, is the turning point in the cycle of creation. If, in this struggle between the expansive (centrifugal) and center-seeking (centripetal) forces, the center-seeking force wins, a resultant force is created that controls all of the factors within the structure. All five factors must be in requisite proportions and the balance of forces within the structure must be such that each factor's energy is controlled and coordinated. The controlling point of all the energies within a structure is called its "vital energy." With vital energy, the evolution of life begins.

## The Creation of Individual Mind

Just as vital energy is the controller of all of the forces within a structure, the vital energy itself must be controlled. Individual ectoplasm, or mind-stuff, emerges to direct the vital energy, controlled by the will of the cosmic mind. Another way of putting this is that the loosening of Shakti's bondage enables the cosmic ectoplasm to reflect, or show through, as individual mind-stuff. Thus begins the second half of the cycle of creation, the attraction of the unit being toward its Self, the supreme consciousness. Matter has evolved from mind, and now mind evolves from matter and moves toward merger with consciousness. The mind-stuff of the individual controls its vital energy through the development of instincts. In the least-developed life forms, the two basic instincts are self-preservation and reproduction.

## EVOLUTION

As reactions are experienced and stored in the mind (a "vibrational record" as it were), behavioral patterns emerge. The entity encounters a clash with its environment, which is recorded in the mind, and the structure evolves capacities for overcoming that clash. Thus more and more complex life forms evolve. The sense of existence emerges in the unit mind, and throughout successive generations the entity develops a more complex nervous and glandular system to control the more highly developed body.

Eventually, from the sense of existence, the ego or the feeling "I act" emerges. The wavelength of the mind becomes more subtle, and ego is formed from a portion of ectoplasm. At this stage, the ego has two functions: determination — or will — and translation into action. Living beings with only mind-stuff act only on mechanical impulses; those with ego as well can make limited decisions about their actions. For example, a worm confronted with a stimulus such as fire can only contract instinctively. An ape, however, when attacked, may either fight or flee. This is due to the more highly developed glandular system and the corresponding development of ego.

## THE HUMAN BEING EMERGES

Moving on in the course of evolution, the mutative tendency begins to wane and the subtle vibration of the sentient tendency carves a place in the individual mind. The subtlest aspect of mind, the sense of self-awareness, awakens. At this stage, the mind of the living being is a complete reflection, potentially, of the mind of God. At last a conscious awareness of that reflection is possible, and a desire to know arises. "Who am I?" "Where do I come from?" "Where am I going?" These are the questions that haunt the human

As the longing for the Great increases, the physical body develops certain complexities for an adjustment with higher psychic demands. Hence we find that in creatures having developed sentiments, the physical body is a composite structure of a large number of glands with their peculiar activities. The developed glandular complexity is essential for facing the psychic clashes in subtler spheres.

— P. R. Sarkar

being and that she alone is capable of asking. The attraction of the supreme nucleus, the longing for the infinite, propels us toward self-realization.

During the long process of evolution, the individual soul is propelled through many incarnations, moving up the scale of complexity, eventually embodying a human form. There are three forces of evolution that guide this process and determine the duration and complexity of each structure in each lifetime.

## THE FORCES THAT EVOLVE THE MIND

First there is the force of physical clash by which the lower portion of mind (sometimes called the ectoplasm) is developed. It is the result of contact between mind and matter, and the resultant clash between the subtle and dense vibrations of the two. As each living being struggles with nature to survive, that struggle refines the mind and helps develop higher capacities for survival. As these higher capacities evolve, the mind needs a subtler structure in which to grow and so takes on subtler physical forms. Early humans evolved because of clash with nature. They developed tools, agriculture, mathematics, science, etc., and as they did so, the human body evolved into a more complex form in order to house the more complex and subtle workings of the mind.

The second force of evolution is that by which the ego evolves — we can describe it as "psychic clash." This is the association with other minds and with ideas. As the mind struggles to attune itself to the wavelength of another more highly evolved mind, clash occurs and the mind expands. It is said that often domestic animals who have a lot of contact with humans will embody as humans in the next life. Constant contact with the vibration of the human mind evolves the animal's ego. In order for it to maintain parallelism between the physical and psychic wavelength, a subtler form is necessary. Education is a form of psychic clash that helps to evolve the human ego.

The third type of clash that acts as an evolutionary force is "spiritual clash," by which intuition is developed. This happens only in the later stages of human evolution, when the mind has evolved sufficiently and the longing for the infinite is intense. This is the attraction between the individual mind and the infinite wavelength of supreme consciousness. It creates the tremendous desire and momentum needed to drive the spiritual aspirant to full self-realization.

As the mind evolves, subtler forms are necessary in order for the body's wavelength to maintain a parallel with the mind.

Now you can begin to see the importance of spiritual practices. Yoga postures, food, meditation, right conduct, service, study of spiritual ideas — all of these activities help the body/mind relationship remain in balance as you evolve.

## NEGATIVE EVOLUTION

According to Tantric philosophy, it is possible for humans to de-evolve into other life forms. Our free will is a result of the full evolution of our minds. We have mind-stuff, ego, and self-awareness; we exist, we act to maintain that existence, and we know. We have the capacity to grasp the universal laws with understanding, and we can choose our actions. We are at a critical juncture.

We are attracted by those familiar basic concerns that dominated our existence in animal embodiments — eating, sleeping, procreation, fear. But we also have a sense of greater fulfillment, a dim memory of infinite bliss. Thus many people wander for lifetimes in a state of confusion, vacillating between the pleasures and pains of animal existence and the unknown journey toward higher consciousness. If a human's mind becomes completely dominated by animal-like instinct, she may need to go back, temporarily, to an animal body to fulfill that propensity before taking a human form again.

----

Recommended Reading:

*Up from Eden* by Ken Wilbur

# Chapter Three
# The Psychospiritual Anatomy

*Woman dancing with hair*
*on fire, woman writhing in the*
*cone of orange snakes, flowering*
*into crackling lithe vines*
*Woman…*

— Marge Piercy,
*The Twelve-Spoked Wheel Flashing*

## THE SUBTLE BODY

*L*ong ago, in many primitive cultures, when someone had a disabling disease, it was thought to be the work of a demon who had either projected some object (a dart, a worm, etc.) inside the person's body, or had extracted the patient's soul. The best cure was thought to be trepanning, or making a hole in the person's skull so the evil spirit or object would come out, or the soul would reenter.

Later, as recently as the nineteenth century, healers remained convinced that such diseases could be removed from the body somehow; they cut arteries or applied leeches to the patient's body in hopes of draining the "bad blood." All through history, people have disbelieved or misunderstood that which they could not see. Medical science has been greatly aided by the anatomists who dissected and examined animal and human bodies. We were finally able to grasp, after thousands of years of trial, error, and superstition, the subtler workings of the physical organs. Yoga experts say that we are almost as primitive in our understanding of the human body and mind now as those ancient physicians. We have yet to realize that the physical body is only one layer in the human organism, one layer of mind. There are many subtle organs, of a psychic nature, that have yet to find their way into anatomical textbooks.

Yoga practitioners long ago discovered these subtle anatomical parts through deep meditation. They experimented, they observed, and they discovered a body "beyond the body" — a kind of psychic structure. They found its development essential to spiritual progress. All of the Tantric spiritual practices came out of these discoveries, updated and refined over thousands of years. Yogic physicians of the future will work with the subtle psychic systems as well as our physical organs to help us heal ourselves, to prevent disease, and to correct imbalances that may affect our mental and spiritual well-being. They will look back with horror upon some of the primitive practices of modern medicine; they will probably shake their heads at the astounding ignorance of human beings in our time.

The physical body and the subtle body are interrelated; they have an impact on one another. For example, a blockage or disturbance in one of the psychic centers can affect physical health because the glandular system is intimately associated with and affected by these psychic centers. Similarly, if the glandular system is out of balance, your mental health will be compromised, a disturbance will arise in one or more of the psychic centers, and your meditation will be impaired. As you progress in your meditation, you will have experiences related to the psychospiritual anatomy. Your spiritual practices and higher lessons in meditation will directly involve these subtle systems; it may be helpful to gain a basic understanding of them now.

## KUNDALINI

A prominent aspect of the philosophy and practice of Tantra is Kundalini Yoga — that which brings the dormant spiritual energy in a living being into fruition, to union with its cause — infinite consciousness. According to Tantra, the human structure is a reflection of the universe. The human mind is a reflection, a replica in microcosm, of the cosmic mind.

In the cycle of creation, as you recall, there is a point at the "top" of the cycle, where consciousness is infinite, both within and beyond everything. There is also a point at the "bottom" of the cycle, where the force of static Shakti exerts the most influence possible — the densest expression of consciousness. It is at this densest point when evolution, as we know it, begins.

So, too, in the human structure, the evolution of the spirit begins at the densest point, at the base of the spine. This point is known as *kula*, meaning "container." Within this container is the *kundalini* or the dormant force of spiritual energy, the expression of cosmic energy in human form. This cosmic energy lies asleep within your psychophysical structure. All spiritual practices strive to awaken this dormant force and to elevate it to oneness with infinite consciousness — the "top" of the cycle — represented in the human structure as the top of the head, the "crown center."

Imagine you are sleeping soundly. Perhaps you have been on a long journey and you haven't slept in a couple of days. Your sleep is so deep you don't notice people going in and out of the room, the sun shining in the window in the morning, the sound of the busy street outside. Then suddenly your alarm clock rings near your ear. It's time to catch your plane home. It takes a special instrument — an alarm, a friend nudging you, a telephone ringing nearby — to awaken you from such a deep slumber.

The kundalini has been sleeping deep inside the kula for eons, since the beginning of evolution. It takes a very special instrument to awaken it. One instrument designed to awaken the kundalini is the *mantra*, a sound vibration repeated in the mind during meditation. It is the key that unlocks the infinite energy residing in every human being and that propels you toward the infinite bliss of self-realization.

A mantra can be especially effective if it has been invested with the tremendous experience of a teacher who has already achieved what you seek. When a mantra is given correctly at the moment of the initial instruction, its vibration awakens the kundalini. Each time it is repeated in the mind, it vibrates the primordial spiritual energy and the kundalini rises. When repetition stops, it returns again to the kula. It is said that the kundalini, when seen with the "inner eye," is as bright as ten million flashes of lightning but as soothing to gaze upon as ten million moons.

Meditation alone, even without the guidance of a teacher, can also awaken the kundalini. It rises through a "psychic canal," the *susumna*, passing through each of the subtler energy centers. The susumna is like the information superhighway, an invisible channel for energy, connecting the subtle energy centers (*chakras*) to the body through a vibrational relationship to the nerves and endocrine system. As the kundalini rises, the practitioner experiences profound states of blissful consciousness, until a total merger with infinite consciousness is attained when the kundalini energy reaches the topmost center, associated with the pineal gland. You may sense the movement of the kundalini, you may not. You will probably not notice anything unusual until much later, after many months or years of meditation. At that time, glimpses of the forces at work in meditation are taken in stride and are actually paid no heed. The goal of unqualified union with the infinite is firmly implanted, and the experiences along the path are merely signs, like markers on a hiking trail.

## CHAKRAS

Remember, for a moment, our discussion of the cycle of creation in the previous chapter. You recall that everything in the universe is composed of the five fundamental factors — solid, liquid, luminous, aerial, and etheric. In the living being, these five factors are controlled by the vital energy, which in turn is controlled by the mind. The five factors in the body are controlled by energy centers along the route of the kundalini. These are called *chakras* or vortexes of psychic energy.

Yoga science links the glandular system with these subtle energy centers. There are seven main chakras, each with its own shape, color, sound vibration, and relationship to the body and mind. The chakra system is a subtle spiritual anatomy that is closely related to the physical body. It links that which is "you" to your mind and body.

The word chakra means wheel or spiral, a fundamental structure in our universe. Think of spiral galaxies, round planets, suns and moons in orbit. Think of the concentric circles of growth in tree trunks, of seashells, of the nautilus with its many-chambered spiral. Think of coiled serpents, cats circling and sleeping in spiral shapes, the opening flower in spring, spiral bales of hay at harvest time, the concentric shapes of snowflakes. The chakra is the wheel, the shape of a container, a spiral path up a mountain. The powerful forces of nature are spiral vortexes: hurricanes, tornados, cyclones, even volcanos. Chakras are fundamental structures in nature that provide the link between spirit and matter; they are multidimensional paradigms of consciousness.

The chakras regulate the subtle energy within the body. There are seven basic chakras, each associated with states of consciousness. They are the containers of psychic propensities or instincts: the longings, desires, and emotions that must be harnessed along the way. The chakras are the controlling points of all the vital elements in your being — physical, emotional, mental, and spiritual. They are closely associated with the endocrine system, and thus have an impact upon your physical and emotional well-being. Spiritually, the chakras are the stepping stones to attainment. The control of each chakra brings more profound states of consciousness and corresponding control over all the forces in the universe. The chakras are the gateways to oneness with the Supreme.

Think of the significance of the number seven. The seven colors of our rainbow, seven notes in the Western musical scale, seven days in a week. The Cabalistic Tree of Life has seven levels. There are seven sacraments in the Christian tradition. Mystic traditions and astrology teach what researchers are now exploring: that human beings go through major life cycles of seven years each.

You may have seen charts that connect the chakras to the colors of the rainbow and the notes of the Western musical scale. However, the number seven may be the only thing they actually have in common. People who have not been trained or have not experienced the vibration, form, and color of the chakras have conveniently, but wrongly, made these associations. Artistically, and perhaps in the field of color therapy, an association can be made between the seven chakras and the colors of the rainbow. But the inherent "color" is quite different and can only be perceived with spiritual insight, not seen by the external eye. Each chakra also has its acoustic root or sound, again, perceived rather than heard, and within each chakra, each mental tendency has its own vibration.

Virtually every spiritual tradition refers to the chakras in some way. Saint John wrote of the "seven spirits before the throne" and the "seven seals on the back of the Book of Life." Other early Christians are said to have used the term "seven churches in Asia." The Tibetans call them "Khor-lo"; the Hopi, in their creation story, speak of energy centers; the early alchemists spoke of seven metals by which crude matter was transmuted into "gold."

## THE VRTTIS

Clustered around each chakra are the *vrttis,* or the mental tendencies that are controlled by that chakra and its relationship to associated physical glands. An increase or decrease or an imbalance in glandular secretions can make the vrttis more or less active. Yoga postures can help balance and regulate the activity of the chakras and thus the glands and vrttis.

According to yoga science, the mind stores reactive "momenta" — the plural of momentum — or *samskaras,* a type of energy created by desire. Some people call it "karma," though technically *karma* means the reaction you experience as a *result* of your reactive momentum. Samskaras are like deposits you make in a bank, to be withdrawn at a later date. They can be inborn, such as the child prodigy who is born with the samskara for musical genius; they can be imposed by parents or society; or they can be acquired throughout life. Everyone has a vastly different set of samskaras, constantly ripening and being expressed. What you think, say, and do, according to yoga philosophy, comes back to you.

According to your particular set of reactive momenta, vrttis are formed; their expression and control depend upon the chakras. The chakras vibrate according to the reactive momenta, and their vibrational expression causes hormones to be secreted. These hormones affect your mental state and thus your actions and reactions. When you can control the chakras, you control the expression of these mental tendencies. You are no longer pulled here and there, tossed about on a sea of emotions, desires, fears, and aversions. Your mind achieves a state of equilibrium in which your samskaras can be expressed in a healthy way and released. Control of the chakras — and thus the glandular secretions and finally the mind — is the object of many meditation practices and yoga postures.

The process of controlling the chakras, and thus the vrttis and physical glands, was invented by yoga master Astavarka in India over 2000 years ago. He called this process "Rajadhiraja Yoga," and taught the system in the area of Bengal, India. Later, the sage Patanjali organized a system he called "Raja Yoga," which included an eight-fold process of holistic health and self-realization. These are not sequential steps, but components of a holistic approach to spiritual development:

(1) *Yama* (ethical behavior): kindness, honesty, responsibility, unity, simplicity.

(2) *Niyama* (spiritual behavior): clarity, acceptance, sacrifice, understanding, spirituality.

(3) *Asanas* (yoga postures).

(4) *Pranayama* (control of the breath).

(5) *Pratyahara* (withdrawing the mind from the physical world).

(6) *Dharana* (intense concentration).

(7) *Dhyana* (true meditation).

(8) *Samadhi* (communion with the Deep Self or Supreme Consciousness).

## THE WHOLE SYSTEM

In yoga, all of the systems of the body, the mind, and the spirit are seen as a whole, inextricably linked, each with its part to play in the daily destiny of human beings. None can be affected exclusively; any impact on one part of any of these systems affects each of the others. In this spirit of wholeness, let's look at the chakras and all of the activity connected with them.

## THE FIRST CHAKRA

The first chakra is located at the base of the perineum. It controls the solid factor of the body and is related to the excretory functions. It is controlled by the conscious layer of mind. It is here where the spiritual and evolutionary journey begins; this is the densest expression of creation, where consciousness, both in the macrocosmic universe and in the microcosmic reflection of mind in the individual, has been solidified to the greatest degree. It is here that the static energy of kundalini, the latent force of cosmic energy in the individual, resides.

When the kundalini awakens, you realize "Brahma exists" — a state associated with this psychic center. This realization is one of great joy. It is not an intellectual process but a state of consciousness in which you sense your oneness with infinite consciousness. You suddenly realize that God is real and exists within your reach, in the core of your own being.

### First Chakra: *Muladhara*

**Meaning:** root

**Shape:** square

**Color:** golden

**Acoustic root:** lam (pronounced "lung")

**Called:** the root chakra, terranian plexus

**Location:** the lowest point of the last bone of the spinal column

**Element:** earth

**Factor:** solid

**Vrttis:** spiritual aspiration, psychospiritual longing, psychic desire, physical lust

**Physical malfunction:** constipation, sciatica, hemorrhoids, obesity, anorexia

**Psychological issues:** survival, ambition, will to live

**Controlled by:** conscious layer of mind

**Body function:** excretory

**Glands:** gonads (ovaries, testes)

**Activities to strengthen:** "grounding" exercises such as Body Level, (p. 90); yoga posture *Yogamudra* (p. 95)

**Foods to strengthen:** proteins in the form of grains, beans, and dairy products

**Color therapy to strengthen:** red

## THE SECOND CHAKRA

The second chakra is located a little higher, at the base of the pelvis. It controls the liquid factor of the body, is related to the sexual functions, and is controlled by the subconscious layer of mind. As the kundalini pierces this chakra, you realize "Brahma is everywhere, Brahma is all that exists."

### Second Chakra: *Svadhisthana*

**Meaning:** sweet

**Shape:** crescent

**Color:** milky white

**Acoustic root:** vam (pronounced "wung")

**Called:** fluidal plexus

**Location:** spinal cord, directly behind root of the genitals

**Element:** water

**Factor:** liquid

**Vrttis:** indifference, lack of common sense, fear of death, lack of confidence, hopelessness, crude behavior

**Physical malfunction:** impotence, kidney and bladder infections, reproductive problems

**Psychological issues:** sexuality, sexual identity, ethics, body image

**Controlled by:** subconscious layer of mind

**Body function:** sexual

**Glands:** gonads (ovaries, testes)

**Activities to strengthen:** yoga postures *Yogamudra* (p. 95) and *Diirgha Pranam* (p. 96); meditation in conjunction with sexual abstinence

**Foods to strengthen:** liquids, especially herbal teas and soups; watery

43

vegetables such as jicama and celery; neem leaves
**Color therapy to strengthen:** orange

A weakness in the first and second chakras can cause psychic distur-
bances that have to do with survival concerns, desires and drives that are "out
of control," and self-image problems. Imbalanced secretion of the associated
glands may cause cruelty and/or narrow-mindedness.

## THE THIRD CHAKRA

Located at the navel point, the third chakra is the controlling point for
the luminous factor — the fiery energy of the body — and is associated with
digestion. It is controlled by the supramental, or intuitive layer of the mind.
You experience the close proximity of your goal as you gain control over this
chakra. You can hardly remember a time when the intense desire for self-realization was not the pivot of your life.

**Third Chakra:** *Manipura*
**Meaning:** fiery gem
**Shape:** triangular
**Color:** fiery red-orange
**Acoustic root:** ram (pronounced "rung")
**Called:** igneous or solar plexus (because of its relatioships with effects of the
sun on the body)
**Location:** at the navel
**Element:** fire
**Factor:** luminous

**Vrttis:** shyness, sadistic tendencies, envy, inertia, melancholy, peevishness, yearning for acquisition, blind attachment, hatred, fear
**Physical malfunctions:** ulcers, pancreatitis, diabetes
**Psychological issues:** personal power, self-esteem, work
**Controlled by:** supramental layer of mind
**Body function:** digestion
**Glands:** pancreas, adrenals
**Activities to strengthen:** yoga postures *Cobra* (p. 96) and *Yogamudra* (p. 95); abdominal crunches; martial arts
**Foods to strengthen:** starches such as potatoes and yams
**Color therapy to strengthen:** yellow

The third chakra is closely connected with intense emotions, with energy, with stress management, and with the functions of the adrenals and the pancreas. It is also an energy center for the sensitive fourth chakra. A weakness in the third chakra causes intense shyness and a fear of speaking in public. Excessive fear builds tension around the third chakra, blocking energy to the fourth chakra and causing heart problems. Strengthening and stabilizing the third chakra can have a profound positive effect on your immune system, your emotional health, and your resilience. In particular, the yoga poses *Yogamudra* (p. 95) and *Cobra* (p. 96), and the practice of *Kaoshikii* (p. 110) can help with problems of fear (ranging from shyness to anxiety and panic), the emotion that most weakens the third chakra and blocks the fourth.

The third chakra is the center of heat for the entire body and is also associated with the liver, the storehouse of the body's heat in the form of energy. When the body is cremated, this area is the last to burn, as it requires a much higher temperature to be destroyed. People often refer to the third chakra as the solar plexus.

## THE FOURTH CHAKRA

Located at the center of the chest, the fourth chakra controls the aerial factor of the body and is related to the body's respiratory and circulatory functions. It is controlled by the subliminal layer of mind. The state of consciousness experienced as the kundalini pierces it is one of divine love. The fourth chakra is often called the "yogic heart" because as the practitioner's attainment rises to this level, she becomes more and more like a lover on fire with devotion to her Beloved. The desires for the experiences, joys, and pleasures of the physical world pale in comparison to the ecstatic, encompassing love your meditation brings. Even the contemplation of the infinite gives you an intense joy that brings a special radiance and grace.

**Fourth Chakra: *Anahata***

**Meaning:** pure, untarnished

**Shape:** circular

**Color:** smoky gray

**Acoustic root:** yam (pronounced "yung")

**Called:** lunar plexus (because of its relationship with effects of the moon on the body)

**Location:** at the center of the chest, just above the sternum

**Element:** air

**Factor:** aerial

**Vrttis:** hope, love, anxiety, depression, helplessness, the effort to arouse

potential, conscience, conceit, avarice, hypocrisy, argumentativeness, remorse
**Physical malfunctions:** heart disease, high blood pressure, asthma
**Psychological issues:** feeling your emotions, joy and pain, gratitude, grief, love, transformation of personal love to universal love, feeling "at one" with others and the universe (attunement)
**Controlled by:** subliminal layer of mind
**Body function:** heart and lungs, circulation and breathing
**Glands:** thymus
**Activities to strengthen:** yoga posture *Cobra* (p. 96); deep meditation, regulated breathing (p. 82); loving kindness in thought, word, and deed; spending time in forests and near natural water sources
**Foods to strengthen:** pure water and air, blue-green algae, chlorella, spirulina, seaweed
**Color therapy to strengthen:** green

It is said that light from the sun and moon affects the body and mind through the "lunar plexus," the container of the fourth chakra. Therefore, light or color therapy is best used on this area.

We can see how the third and fourth chakras are related through the thymus gland. Chronic stress caused by unrelenting tension or negative emotions causes tension in the third chakra and pushes the adrenals into action. Steroids from the adrenals act on the thymus, at the fourth chakra, causing the destruction of T-cells, disabling the immune system. Thus someone can literally die of a "broken heart."

Negative experiences that affect us at the "heart" level can weaken this chakra. Other expressions we use in our intuitive understanding of this chakra's function include: "heartfelt thanks," "from my heart," "my heart sank," "it broke my heart," and "have a heart."

## THE FIFTH CHAKRA

Located at the throat, this chakra controls the etheric factor and is related to the function of speech. It is controlled by the highest layer of mind, the subtle causal layer. This chakra controls the ones below, thus it coordinates all the energies of the physical body. Control of this chakra brings with it the knowledge of past, present, and future. You hear the cosmic sound, the Aunkara ("AUM") in deep meditation. You are one with the cosmic mind, from whom the creation ("A" sound), the operation ("U"), and the destruction ("M") of the entire cosmos resides. You are merged with the pure "I am" — the origin of the universe.

### Fifth Chakra: *Vishuddha*

**Meaning:** purification
**Shape:** hexagonal
**Color:** rainbow hued
**Acoustic root:** ham (pronounced "hung")
**Called:** sidereal plexus
**Location:** throat (at vocal chord)
**Element:** ether
**Factor:** etheric
**Vrttis:** some of the vrttis at this chakra are fruition, accomplishment, development of mundane knowledge, integrity, resolve, surrender to the Supreme, attraction, and repulsion

**Physical malfunctions:** colds, sore throats, bronchitis, thyroid and hearing problems

**Psychological issues:** listening, expressing your thoughts and feelings, creative expression

**Controlled by:** subtle causal layer of mind

**Body function:** speech and hearing

**Glands:** thyroid, parathyroid

**Activities to strengthen:** yoga postures *Sarvaungasana* (*Shoulderstand*, p. 107), *Matsyamudra* (*Fish*, p. 108), singing devotional songs, listening to devotional music, creative artistic expression

**Foods to strengthen:** fruits and fruit juices

**Color therapy to strengthen:** blue

Control of this chakra brings with it paranormal experiences such as extrasensory perception and precognition. In deep meditation, the cosmic sound "aum" is heard and the meditator merges with the cosmic mind, within which the creation, preservation, and destruction of the universe resides.

Psychospiritual issues addressed by strengthening this chakra include difficulty in speaking one's mind, expressing oneself artistically, and being able to empathize with others.

For balanced, normal body processes and normal thinking, we need exactly the right amount of thyroid and parathyroid hormones. The yoga poses Shoulderstand (p. 107) and Fish (p. 108) help maintain this perfect balance.

## THE SIXTH CHAKRA

As realization reaches the next two chakras, all objective reality is dissolved. The consciousness of the individual gives way to the universal consciousness, beyond even cosmic mind.

The sixth chakra is called the "seat of mind" and is located at the "third eye," directly above the nose, between the eyebrows. No physical factor is controlled here. Beyond the reach of limitation, having broken the mirror of the ego, when the kundalini reaches this chakra you are merged in the consciousness from which the mind of the Supreme originates.

### Sixth Chakra: *Ajina*

**Meaning:** to see or perceive

**Shape:** triangular

**Color:** none

**Acoustic root:** none

**Called:** third eye

**Location:** at the bridge of the nose, between the eyes

**Element:** none

**Factor:** none

**Vrttis:** mundane knowledge, spiritual knowledge

**Psychological issues:** ideals, beliefs, intuition, self-realization

**Physical malfunctions:** headaches, vision problems, cognitive difficulties

**Controlled by:** atman (soul)

**Body function:** thought, awareness

**Glands:** pituitary

**Activities to strengthen:** yoga postures *Yogamudra* (p. 95), *Diirgha Pranam* (p. 96); study involving concentration; meditation

**Foods to strengthen:** none

**Color therapy to strengthen:** deep blue (indigo)

The sixth chakra is the focus of most meditation practices. Meditation strengthens the functions of this chakra and regulates the pituitary gland. As practice in meditation progresses and powers of concentration develop, the seventh chakra becomes the focus of practice.

## THE SEVENTH CHAKRA

The seventh chakra is known as the "thousand-petaled lotus" because it is the controlling point for every tendency in the individual. It is here that the kundalini reaches its goal and awareness merges completely in infinite consciousness, the origin of origins. There is no human expression for this state. It is beyond anything we can ever imagine. We know of it only by its after-effects: the waves of ecstasy that follow even after a fraction of a moment in that state. When no reactive momenta are left to bind the individual to the physical world, the merger in this state will be complete. Like the doll made of salt who tried to measure the ocean, you merge in the immeasurable expanse of your own origin. This is the goal of human life.

**Seventh Chakra:** *Sahasrara*
**Meaning:** thousand petals
**Shape:** thousand-petaled lotus
**Color:** none
**Acoustic root:** none
**Called:** seat of the soul
**Location:** at the top (crown) of the head

**Element:** none
**Factor:** none
***Vrttis:*** none
**Physical malfunctions:** none
**Psychological issues:** none
**Controlled by:** universal consciousness
**Body function:** none
**Glands:** pineal
**Activities to strengthen:** deep meditation
**Foods to strengthen:** none
**Color therapy to strengthen:** violet

This chakra controls the one thousand expressions of all the vrttis. When consciousness reaches this chakra in deep meditation, complete absorption (*samadhi*) is attained.

## THE LAYERS OF THE MIND

Yoga science says that the body is composed of the five fundamental factors — solid, liquid, luminous, aerial, etherial — which make up the entire universe and are controlled by the mind. The mind is composed of five layers (conscious, subconscious, supramental, subliminal, and subtle causal) plus its container, the physical body. The mind controls the chakras, and thus the expression of the vrttis, or mental tendencies.

Existence is a continuum, moving from the crude, dense expression of consciousness to the subtle, and then to the unity of infinite consciousness, where all is one. Along this continuum are several layers, wherein the expression of consciousness in the form of body and mind performs the functions that are necessary to maintain individual existence and progress. The layers of the mind are called the *kosas* (pronounced "koh-shas"). On the following pages, you can see how each functions and how each is developed. The spiritual practices, including yoga postures, meditation, exercise, and regulation of the diet all contribute to the holistic development of all the layers of the mind.

## THE PHYSICAL BODY
**Sanskrit name:** *Annamaya Kosa* ("made of food")
**Dominating tendency:** static
**Function:** mechanical
**Controlled by:** conscious mind
**Naturally developed by:** physical labor, exercise, balanced diet
**Spiritual practices that develop it:** yoga postures

## CONSCIOUS LAYER
**Sanskrit name:** *Kamamaya Kosa* ("desire")
**Dominating tendency:** static
**Function:** sensing, through sensory organs; desire or aversion; acting through motor organs
**Controls:** first chakra
**Naturally developed by:** the struggle for existence
**Spiritual practices that develop it:** right conduct (Yama and Niyama, p. 139)

53

The conscious mind functions through the senses, desire or aversion, and acts through the motor organs. On this level of mind, we perform all the functions that make us similar to animals: we eat, we sleep, we procreate, and we react to our environment.

## SUBCONSCIOUS LAYER

**Sanskrit name:** *Manomaya Kosa* ("mental")
**Dominating tendency:** mutative
**Function:** controls conscious mind, memory, contemplation, experience of pleasure and pain, dreams
**Controls:** second chakra
**Naturally developed by:** the struggle for existence, thinking, remembering, reacting
**Spiritual practices that develop it:** control of breath (*Pranayama*)

The subconscious mind functions through memory, contemplation, the experience of pleasure and pain, and dreams. The vast majority of most people's thought processes go on at this level. It is the layer of information management, computation, philosophy, and memory.

According to yoga, memory has two functions. *Cerebral memory* computes and stores information on a deeper level than our conscious awareness. This is the part of our mind that is aware of every detail of our environment and experience. Learning specialists are now beginning to tap the potential of this underground warehouse of experience. In Bulgaria, a lot of research has been done on a new system of learning they call "suggestopedia" or "super-learning." Using music and deep relaxation to occupy the conscious mind with certain rhythms that make it calm and receptive, information is repeated and seems to be absorbed directly at the subconscious level. Often, students are able to learn a year's worth of material in one month.

*Extra-cerebral memory* is as yet unproven by modern science. It is a level of mind experienced by practiced meditators and people with paranormal abilities; it seems to be a memory bank that is somehow beyond the brain. Memories of past-life experiences come from this part of the mind.

## SUPRAMENTAL LAYER

**Sanskrit name:** *Atimanasa Kosa* ("higher mind")
**Dominating tendency:** mutative
**Function:** creative insight, intuition, paranormal phenomena; the "all-knowing" layer
**Controls:** third chakra
**Naturally developed by:** education, new environments, contact with more highly developed minds
**Spiritual practices that develop it:** sense withdrawal in meditation

The supramental mind functions through creative insight, intuition, paranormal phenomena (extrasensory perception, precognition, telepathy, telekinesis, etc.) and acts as a storehouse of knowledge of the past, present, and future. This is the level of mind from which we begin to experience "oneness" with what we may call the Cosmic Mind. We tap into it sometimes when we have a moving experience in nature, or through art or music, or a "peak" experience that takes us beyond our normal awareness.

Psychologist Abraham Maslow, the founder of the transpersonal and

*Those who are truly nonattached do not deny life, they embrace it, for they feel the touch of the eternal hidden within all the changing forms of their lives. They become like the child who is overjoyed to receive a new dress from her mother; one minute she caresses and hugs it to her, and the next, when she finds a beautiful toy, she leaves the dress to embrace the toy. Later she drops the toy to run after a flower – she is attached to nothing. So those who see all objects and creatures of the world as radiant waves in the ocean of universal consciousness and deal with them without attachment or aversion, enjoy inexhaustible bliss, for they are in love with the Infinite.*

— Avtk. Ananda Mitra Ac.,
*Beyond the Superconscious Mind*

humanist movements in psychology, knew that a level existed beyond what is normally experienced, and spent his life studying it. He decided that, rather than studying people who were mentally ill, he would study "self-actualizers," people who had fulfilling lives and who were perceived to be courageous, creative, humble, and relatively free from anxiety. By showing us the qualities possessed by these extraordinary people, he pointed the way to health and integration, and gave us a new way of perceiving the potential of every human being.

This is the layer of mind through which we experience insight, creative flashes, and "Aha!" realizations. It seems to be reached through a balance of concentration and relaxation, and a depth of spirit that seeks unity and understanding beyond daily experience. Some people seem to be born with paranormal faculties, regularly (and sometimes uncontrollably) dipping into this layer of the mind and experiencing psychic phenomenon such as premonitions and extrasensory perception. Yoga philosophy says that this level of mind is accessible to all and is reached as a matter of course through meditation practice. Human beings of the future will think these experiences are perfectly normal and will learn how to use this layer of the mind for individual and societal benefit. This layer is also known as the first layer of the Superconscious Mind.

## SUBLIMINAL LAYER
**Sanskrit name:** *Vijinanamaya Kosa* ("special knowledge")
**Dominating tendency:** sentient
**Function:** discrimination and detachment
**Controls:** fourth chakra

**Naturally developed by:** contact with human beings who are more mentally and spiritually advanced, education

**Spiritual practices that develop it:** concentration, meditation

The subliminal mind functions through the faculties of discrimination and detachment. This layer is reached early in life only by a few deeply spiritual people; it becomes more accessible to the yoga practitioner with deep meditation and as we age. It is the place from which we begin to understand the relativity of our bodies and the world around us. The qualities of gentleness, patience, serenity, humility, and broad-mindedness develop as this layer unfolds.

## SUBTLE CAUSAL LAYER

**Sanskrit name:** *Hiranyamaya Kosa* ("golden")

**Dominating tendency:** sentient

**Function:** yearning for self-realization

**Controls:** fifth chakra

**Naturally developed by:** attraction to God, desiring of limitlessness

**Spiritual practices that develop it:** deep devotional meditation

The subtle causal mind has one function: the yearning for self-realization. This is the thin veil of the mind that separates it from merging with Infinite Consciousness. When we have access to this layer of mind, we are firmly established in universalism; we can no longer make divisions and judgements about others and the world, for we feel that we are a part of every atom of the universe and that the scope of our love is truly infinite.

Thus yogis have always emphasized the importance of the gradual and careful preparation of the mind and body to receive and control the unlimited powers of the superconscious state. One master told his disciple, who had begged him to give him the experience of higher consciousness, "As a small lamp bulb would be shattered by excessive voltage, so your nerves are unready for the cosmic current. If I gave you the infinite ecstasy right now, you would burn as though every cell were on fire." Through centuries of experimentation, a scientific physical and mental system was developed to safely and easily attain the bliss of higher consciousness and then integrate these expanded states with normal, waking consciousness, to live life with fuller awareness.

— Avtk. Ananda Mitra Ac., *Beyond the Superconscious Mind*

In summary, the body is composed of the five fundamental factors, which are controlled by the mind. The five layers of mind control, through the vital energy, each of the lower chakras respectively. The fifth chakra, however, is the controlling point for all of these. Spiritual practices such as meditation in its various forms, yoga postures, and right conduct develop each of these systems. When you are able to gain access to the higher layers of mind, you will have the concentration to control, develop, and strengthen the chakras and the bodily functions, leading to greater mental clarity, emotional stability, and physical longevity.

As the body becomes more refined, the chakras are purified, strengthened, and controlled. Refining the body helps you reach the higher layers of mind. Tantra is holistic in that it recognizes the interconnectedness and interdependence of body, mind, and spirit. You cannot attain enlightenment merely by doing yoga postures; you will not if you neglect the body, for at some point the unrefined body will not be able to handle the subtlety of mind, and it will break down.

## PSYCHIC POWERS

As each chakra is controlled — through the intense effort in meditation and spiritual practices that develop the higher layers of mind — you attain access to the infinite storehouse of power and knowledge that we call "cosmic mind."

The highly advanced practitioner may develop the ability to levitate, to walk on water, to make things appear and disappear, to infuse fragrance in objects, to cure diseases, and any number of other "supernatural" powers. Because the chakras are the controlling points for the fundamental factors, control of each of these also gives the yogi access to the manipulation of matter. But she knows that such powers are dangerous playthings. Great masters may occasionally use these powers to illustrate some aspect of their teachings to their students. But the greatest masters always point out the dangers of these powers and encourage their students to disregard them and keep moving straight toward their goal.

The deeper levels of the mind are accessible to all of us; extrasensory perception, precognition, intuition, creative insight, etc., are abilities we all possess. Intense concentration, drugs, or altered consciousness from a shock will often temporarily elevate us to a higher dimension. Some people, because of intense concentration in a previous life, are born with "supernatural" abilities. But without the regular practice of deep meditation performed with the goal of infinite expansion, these abilities can bring more pain than pleasure. Inspiration from the superconscious mind, without the discrimination instilled by meditation, must filter through the subconscious mind and can thus become confused with limited sense impressions. The person possessing these abilities not only develops a false sense of power and prestige, but her "guidance" may adversely impact the lives of people she encounters.

Artistic and scientific geniuses often work in a state of superconscious awareness, which they then have difficulty integrating into their everyday consciousness — a difficulty that has sometimes led to disorientation, and even madness or suicide. There is little to be gained by hankering after occult powers. Most of us, however, are a long way from having to be mindful of their dangers. With regular practice you will gradually notice a sharpening of your senses, a keener awareness of the things and people around you, an intuitive insight that you may not have had access to before, and a deepening respect for the unlimited potential of the human mind.

Recommended Reading:

*Roots of Consciousness* by Jeffrey Mishlove

*Wheels of Life* by Anodea Judith

*Yoga Psychology* by Swami Abhedananda

*Yoga Psychology* by P. R. Sarkar

# Chapter Four
# Physical Health

*The Spirit of the Fountain dies not.*
*It is called the Mysterious Feminine.*
*The Doorway of the Mysterious Feminine*
*Is called the Root of Heaven-and-Earth.*

*Lingering like gossamer, it has only a hint of existence;*
*And yet when you draw upon it, it is inexhaustible.*

— Lao Tzu

## A BALANCED APPROACH

Now it's time to learn about the things you can do to help develop all these different aspects of yourself. I will cover some of the practices that can help you do this and then suggest a starting point. It is important to go slowly. Don't try to do everything at once, or you will soon be frustrated.

In order to develop yourself on deeper levels, you'll want to be sure your body is fit and that you know what to do to keep it that way. Certain practices are very conducive to meditation, and you'll want to cut down on or avoid some things in order to make your meditation easy, your body more comfortable, and to keep your emotions in balance. For example, a diet heavy in meat and rich foods, cigarette smoking, and alcohol consumption can interfere with your concentration and damage your health. You may wish to experiment with cutting down or eliminating some of these and see if your meditation, mental balance, and physical health are affected in any way.

Design your daily program with all-around equilibrium in mind. What must you do to keep your life in balance? This will change as you grow. For example, when you go through phases of longer and more intensive meditation sessions, you'll also want to pay attention to dietary, environmental, and physical changes that will help you maintain a sense of equilibrium. Doing a lot of meditation without developing the other aspects of your being can have harmful effects. The physical, mental, and spiritual aspects of your existence all emit their particular vibrational expressions. The harmonious rhythm of these is called "health." If one thing changes and the others don't, the lack of parallelism can cause physical or even mental illness.

## THE PHYSIOLOGICAL BENEFITS OF YOGA POSTURES

Thousands of years ago, yogis meditating deep in jungles carefully observed the wild animals who shared their solitude. They began to detect the techniques that nature gives less evolved creatures to keep them healthy, agile, and alert. They watched how different animals instinctively cured themselves and began to experiment with these animal postures upon their own bodies. After long and intensive study, practice, and adjustment, they created a systematic series of physical postures known as *asanas*. Many yoga postures are named for the animals that inspired them: cobra, lion, peacock, fish.

Yoga postures balance the glandular secretions, relax and tone the muscles and nervous system, stimulate circulation, oxygenate the blood, stretch stiff ligaments and tendons, limber joints, massage internal organs, align the spine, and calm and concentrate the mind.

The entire body is controlled by hormones. The twisting and bending positions of yoga postures, held for particular periods of time, place continued and specific pressure upon the various endocrine glands, thus regulating their secretions. The endocrine system is intimately related to our emotions. Over-secretion of certain hormones can cause a wide range of emotional imbalances; premenstrual syndrome is a good example of this.

You feel emotions in your body: When you are angry, you might say, "My blood is boiling!" When sad, you have a "lump in the throat." Fear makes "butterflies in the stomach." When disappointed, you say, "My heart sank." You can control, to a great extent, your emotional reaction to various kinds of stress by controlling the glandular secretions through yoga postures.

## THE MUSCLES AND LIGAMENTS

As opposed to the rapid, vigorous contraction of muscles during aerobic exercise, yoga postures involve slow, sustained contraction and/or stretching of muscle groups. This movement is then held, in a state of relaxation, for a specified period of time: the time it takes to comfortably pause between breaths (a count of eight). During this pause, circulation to the area is enhanced and muscles relax more deeply than during sleep. Energy is accumulated rather than depleted, and the practitioner feels relaxed and refreshed.

Yoga postures involve many groups of muscles that are not ordinarily exercised through aerobics or sports. A thorough session of postures — lasting thirty to forty minutes — will contract, stretch, and release virtually every muscle in the body, toning the entire muscular system, increasing circulation, and oxygenating the blood without causing strain or pain.

Yoga postures perfectly utilize all of the factors necessary for efficient muscular activity, including stretching, warmth, and viscosity. By warming and stretching a muscle before contraction, its efficiency is vastly increased. Athletes are trained to "warm up" with deep breathing (which oxygenates the blood, increasing circulation and warmth to the muscles) and easy stretches.

The faster muscles are contracted, the less efficiently they work. The slow, sustained stretches and deep breathing involved in yoga postures create the perfect situation for efficient muscle use and development.

The ligaments — bands of fibrous tissues that connect the bones and other structures — tend to tighten and shorten with age and disuse. Thus, poor posture and lack of exercise can lead to stiffness and discomfort. Even athletes who daily exercise their muscles can become stiff and inflexible, and thus more prone to injury, without an awareness of the need to stretch and nourish (via deep circulation) the muscles and ligaments.

## THE SPINE

The spine is composed of thirty-three vertebrae (bony "links") separated by cushions, or discs, the body's shock absorbers. With the continual upright pounding involved in our daily activities (walking, running, sitting, lifting), these cushions can become compressed. The flexibility of the spine is reduced and more of the shock is absorbed by the musculature, causing fatigue and finally, an aching pain. Yoga postures stretch the spine and send circulation through these important areas, thus reconditioning the vertebral column and allowing the discs to return to their normal, springy function.

The spinal cord, which is literally an extension of the brain into the body, runs through holes in each vertebra. The spinal cord has nerves running in and out of it between every two vertebrae. These nerves control many of the sensory and motor functions of the entire body. The muscles of the spinal column are also paired, and if one of the pair is weakened by poor posture or stress, the strong one is likely to pull the vertebrae out of alignment. While chiropractic or other healing modalities may help to realign the spine, if the weakened condition of the muscle persists, the strained condition will return. Yoga postures can elongate and align the spine, strengthen the muscles, and limber the ligaments that distribute our activity and energy along its axis.

The spine is divided into five groups of vertebrae. The *cervical* vertebrae provide support for the ever-mobile head; this group must be highly flexible, and is vulnerable to injury. It is important to keep this group aligned and nourished with blood flow and movement. The *thoracic* group is larger and more rigid; this group gives support to the ribs and chest to make breathing possible. The third group, the *lumbar,* must combine strength to support the upper body with flexibility to permit the movements of bending and twisting; because of this flexibility, this is also a vulnerable group. The fourth group is the *sacral* or pelvic group, which begins life as separate vertebrae but during the first months in the womb, fuses into a single bone. The last group is the *coccygeal* — commonly known as the "tailbone."

Yoga postures are designed to stretch the anterior and posterior longitudinal ligaments, which connect all these vertebrae. When these ligaments

are flexible, the spine maintains the right curvature of each group of vertebrae, and the spongy discs are flexible and able to absorb energy, which is
then distributed healthily throughout the system, sort of like the lightning
rod grounds and diffuses the electricity from a lightning strike. When these
ligaments become shortened and rigid, all kinds of problems can arise. The
shocks are not absorbed well by discs that are flattened; more stress is then put
on the muscles and ligaments, which can pull the spine out of alignment,
compress nerves, and cause pain and injury.

## THE JOINTS

Babies move with an incredible range of motion. Many of the yoga postures we teach our bodies to adopt are inherent in the natural movements of
an infant. As the child grows, the flexible cartilage is gradually replaced by
bone, as new bone is deposited again and again around the circumference of
the cartilage; this growth continues until early adulthood. During this period,
we are attuned to the natural rhythms of our bodies as we stretch, play, reach,
bend, sit, squat, crawl, and tumble head over heels with glee! Children don't
need to do yoga postures because their lives are one long yoga session. But as
we reach adulthood and our bones harden to their final level, a daily yoga session can keep our bodies as flexible and easygoing as they are in childhood.

The joints provide places for the ligaments, tendons, and muscles to
attach and thus are pivotally important to our flexibility. Due to poor posture,
sitting repeatedly in chairs with the head and neck thrust forward, and lack of
movement, our ligaments begin to shorten and stiffen and to limit the flexibility of the joints. Movement becomes tight and painful. Even athletes can
experience this stiffening, if athletic activity is limited to one range of

motions, and involves little stretching and slow movement of the entire body.

Yoga provides exactly the type of movement that keeps the joints "oiled," the ligaments flexible, and the muscles toned and strong. A daily routine of yoga postures keeps our bodies young and supple. Deep circulation to the joints is enhanced, and awareness causes us to move our bodies in the natural, balanced fashion for which they are intended.

## THE CIRCULATION

Yoga postures contribute more than the mechanical stretching of muscles, ligaments, and tendons and the full range of motion of the joints. The deep breathing and held stretches get our blood moving smoothly into all parts of our bodies, increasing the elasticity of our blood vessels and bathing our tissues with nutrients and oxygen.

Some yoga postures (the "reverse" postures such as Shoulderstand, p. 107) benefit the valves that return blood to the heart. During these postures, blood flows back to the heart without effort, reducing normal pressures and giving the valves a rest they would not get even when we are resting or sleeping. Only while performing these postures can the capillary beds (tiny blood vessels) in the legs and feet drain completely, which thoroughly cleanses the tissues.

## THE INTERNAL ORGANS

All of our internal organs get a gentle massage during the practice of yoga postures. The combination of deep, diaphragmatic breathing and the squeezing and stretching of the postures increases circulation into and out of each of the vital organs — heart, lungs, kidneys, liver, spleen, pancreas, stomach, and intestines. Thus the function of our vital organs is enhanced and toxins

The novice in Yoga training feels his or her articulations rapidly becoming agile and easily managed as the training progresses. Since medical pathology is well aware of the tremendous importance of a good articular condition, we can easily realize the enormous advantage obtainable through making the articulations soft with the yoga postures.

—— Steven Brena, M.D.,
*Yoga and Medicine*

are carried away to be excreted. Many of the postures promote digestion, ensuring the quick processing of nutrients and elimination of waste, which is required for optimum health.

## THE PSYCHOPHYSICAL BENEFITS OF YOGA POSTURES

One of the unique features of yoga is that it benefits more than just our physical conditioning. In fact, the main purpose of the practice of yoga postures is not exercise; rather, it is the systematic "innercise" of the endocrine system, which affects the way we think and feel.

Hormones regulate the body processes with extreme precision. Irregularities in the timing or levels of their release can lead to disease and mental imbalance. Yoga postures are thus to be practiced carefully and with great precision for the most benefit. First, let's take a close look at the endocrine system and how it works; then we can better understand how yoga postures affect the secretion of hormones to alter and balance our state of mind.

### THE ENDOCRINE SYSTEM

Our education generally gives us little information on the purpose, function, and importance of our endocrine systems. However, according to yoga science, the glands and their secretions are possibly the most important of all the organs in our bodies, for they are directly linked with the mind and emotions. The glands are the vehicles through which the mind commands and communicates with the body. The immune system is completely dependent upon this communication.

The glands are organs, consisting of specialized tissues, that produce and/or secrete materials essential to body harmony. There are two types of glands. The first type, called *exocrine* glands, are ducts through which secretions pass, including the salivary glands, tear ducts, and the liver. Their secretions go directly to the affected part of the body. The second type are the ductless, or *endocrine*, glands. Secretions from these glands ooze into the bloodstream from cells that make up the glands, then the blood carries the secretions to various parts of the body. The secretions of the endocrine glands are known as *hormones*, chemical substances that control other cells of the body. Endocrinology (the study of hormones) is a rapidly growing science, now merging with neuroscience (the study of the brain and central nervous system). As recently as 1970, only about twenty hormones had been identified; now researchers think there may be as many as two hundred! In this book, we will look at the main glandular functions and their hormones.

The *gonads* are exocrine as well as endocrine glands. The gonads are affected particularly at the time of fetal development, puberty, and menopause. The hormones secreted by these glands include *testosterone* (male testes), and *progesterone* and *estrogens* (female ovaries and corpus leuteum). According to yoga science, imbalanced secretion of these glands causes the psychic tendencies toward cruelty and narrow-mindedness. This is somewhat borne out by Western science. In a study of eighty-nine male prison inmates, Georgia State University social psychologist James R. Dabbs, Jr. found that those with higher concentrations of testosterone had more often been convicted of violent crimes. Since testosterone levels usually peak between the ages of sixteen and eighteen, this finding may help explain why men of that age are on the verge of their most crime-prone years. Testosterone increases the tendency toward aggression and physical activity, and also spurs the sex drive and the capacity to act on it. A testosterone-blocking drug, cyproterone acetate, has been given as an alternative to incarceration for some men found guilty of aberrant sexual behavior and has been effective in bringing that behavior under control in many cases.

The sudden flood of sex hormones is what makes adolescence such a roller-coaster ride. Menstruation, acne, embarrassing erections, and mood swings — all caused by hormones — make life interesting for kids (and their parents!) during this watershed time. The body gears up for its age-old purpose: reproduction and protection of the young.

The *adrenal glands,* located near the kidneys, control sudden bursts of energy in response to danger or stress. They secrete the hormone *adrenalin,* activating what has been called the "flight-or-fight response." An imbalance involving the adrenal glands may be implicated in the conditions of high blood pressure, heart disease, ulcers, depression, and cancer.

The adrenals consist of two parts: the cortex and the medulla. The adrenal cortex has three layers:

(1) The outermost layer (zona glomerulosa) produces the mineral-metabolizing hormone *aldosterone* and exerts an influence on the volume, water balance, and pressure of the bloodstream.

(2) The central layer (zona faciculata) produces *hydrocortisone* and *cortico-sterone*. These control the conversion of proteins to carbohydrates, and influence both the blood sugar level and the glycogen stored in the liver. These hormones act as anti-inflammatory and antiallergic agents by mobilizing cells produced by the thymus gland. Corticosterone, when oversecreted due to stress, suppresses the immune system and is a factor in mental and

emotional disorders such as chronic depression and manic-depressive illness. It is also found in higher than average levels in people who are shy and withdrawn.

(3) The innermost layer (zona reticularis) produces the sex hormones *androgen* and *estrogen*.

The second part of the adrenal body is the medulla, a collection of nerve cells belonging to the sympathetic aspect of the autonomic nervous system. Any extraordinary stimulation — stress, fear, anger, pain, joy, ecstacy — triggers the release of its hormones, *adrenalin* and *noradrenalin*. These stimulate the release of *glycogen* from the liver and cause the heart to beat faster and stronger. Breathing increases to facilitate oxygenation of more blood passing through the lungs.

Another chemical reaction happens when the adrenal medulla is called to action. When adrenalin gets to the brain, it stimulates the hypothalamus to release *CRH* (corticotropin-releasing hormone), which makes the pituitary gland secrete *ACTH* (adrenocorticotropic hormone). The ACTH acts upon the adrenal cortex — which releases corticosteroids from its central layer — increasing blood sugar and speeding up metabolism. All this happens in a flash, and the body is ready to encounter danger if it needs to. This is a wonderful system when it works in a healthy, balanced way. But, if due to diet, upbringing, conditioning, etc., our bodies "learn" to interpret mild events with this reaction, we can get into trouble. Too much ACTH means tension, irritability, fatigue, and a lowered resistance to disease. This faulty interpretation of events is learned, or conditioned, from infancy. An infant whose cries are not responded to must cry ever more intensely to get its needs met. Its body learns to interpret being left alone as abandonment, and the

It is likely that the level of subtle psychological violence perpetrated on children by parents, teachers and other adults who are unconscious of their actions and the effects of these actions on the self-esteem of children far exceeds the epidemic proportions of outright physical and psychological abuse. It influences generation after generation of people in terms of how they feel about themselves and what they conceive of as possible in their lives. We try to compensate in many ways in order to feel God deep in our hearts. But until the wounds are healed rather than covered over and denied, our efforts are not likely to result in wholeness or health. They are more likely to result in disease.

— Richard Gerber,
*Vibrational Medicine*

fear and rage of abandonment flood the body with stress hormones. When this happens over and over again, the body becomes accustomed to these rushes of stress hormones and the stimulus needed to produce them becomes less pronounced. A crying infant is one small example. It is no wonder so many people have so little patience, concentration, and peace of mind as adults; as a matter of course, our bodies are producing mind-altering chemicals at a remarkable rate.

In prehistoric times, the danger that caused the release of adrenaline — confrontation with a bear or lion, perhaps — made sense. We needed all the adrenalin we could get in such a situation, to fight or to flee for our lives. But with the prolonged, unmitigated stresses of our present society, we experience the same release of hormones when caught behind a slow truck in traffic! With no opportunity to fight or flee, and in fact knowing that this stimulus is *not* life-threatening, we simmer and burn, victims of patterns created in childhood and the chemicals they automatically produce in our bodies. Prolonged stress and a constant barrage of stress hormones are involved in a host of problems and diseases, from depression to upper respiratory infections and cancer.

The *pancreas*, located at the upper center of the abdominal area, below the stomach, is intimately involved in the digestion of food and its conversion into energy. Like the gonads, it is both exocrine and endocrine in nature. As food passes from the stomach to the small intestine, pancreatic juices, rich in digestive enzymes, break it down and neutralize the stomach acid. These enzymes convert protein to amino acids, fats to fatty acids and glycerol, and carbohydrates to sugars. These nutrients then travel to the liver for storage and to other parts of the body as they are needed.

The endocrine function of the pancreas regulates blood sugar with the hormones *insulin* and *glucagon*. These hormones act cooperatively to keep the blood sugar level stable. Over- or undersecretion of these hormones can result in diabetes or hypoglycemia. Certain types of chronic stress can inflame the pancreas, causing pancreatitis, a condition of acute pain with vomiting and a complete halt to the digestive process.

The *thymus gland* has two major functions: the promotion of growth and the function of the immune system. The thymus is often referred to as the "gland of childhood" because it is large during childhood and shrinks substantially with growth.

During childhood, the thymus helps regulate all the other endocrine glands and controls growth. After puberty, it stops regulating growth; its remaining function is to influence the immune system through the lymphatic system.

The thymus programs a large number of cells (called *lymphocytes*, found in the blood and lymph) to defend the body. During times of stress, the steroids from the adrenals trigger the expulsion of thymus-derived white cells or *T-cells* from the thymus — cells that define the body's immune response. But if the stress is chronic and negative, the same triggers can cause a negative effect. Certain steroids from the adrenals act on the thymus, causing the destruction of T-cells, thus lowering the ratio of helper to suppressor cells and disabling the immune system.

The *thyroid* is a shield-shaped gland in the neck at the level of the larynx. It secretes *thyroxin* and *triiodothyronine*, which control the body's energy metabolism (the speed at which the body operates). The thyroid is our thermostat, controlling heat, energy, growth, repair, and waste processes.

*E*very time you say something to yourself containing a negative emotional charge, it has a tiny but measurable negative effect on your body.

—— Dennis D. Jaffe,
*Healing from Within*

73

*I* am convinced that unconditional love is the most powerful known stimulant for the immune system. If I told patients to raise their blood levels of immune globulins or killer T-cells, no one would know how. But if I can teach them to love themselves and others fully, the same changes happen automatically. The truth is, love heals.

—Bernie Seigel, M.D.

Thyroid function is necessary for development during puberty and is an important component of mental alertness. A lack of thyroid function can cause a condition known as myxedema, with symptoms of apathy, weight gain, drowsiness, and sensitivity to cold. Overfunctioning of the thyroid can lead to symptoms of nervousness, irritability, weight loss, and fatigue.

There are four *parathyroid* glands, located in the body of the thyroid gland. They are also concerned with metabolism; the parathyroids regulate mineral metabolism, contributing to the calcium/phosphorus balance in the blood and bones. The hormones secreted by the parathyroids are known as *PTH* (parathormone) and *calcitonin*. PTH stimulates the release of calcium from bone, while calcitonin inhibits its release. Blood calcium is important for the nervous system's stability; in the absence of functioning parathyroids, nervous excitability increases as much as a thousand times and can lead to a condition called tetany, and also even to death.

The *pituitary gland* was once known as the "bandmaster of the endocrine orchestra." However, it is now known that the pituitary is controlled by the *hypothalamus*. The pituitary is made up of two types of tissue (located in the anterior and posterior portions of the gland), which have different but complementary functions. It is located in the center of the head at the level of the bridge of the nose and just above the back portion of the roof of the nasal cavity.

The anterior portion of the pituitary relays messages from the hypothalamus to the other endocrine glands. It secretes hormones that activate the other endocrine glands: ACTH activates the adrenal glands; *TSH* (thyroid-stimulating hormone) activates the thyroid; *gonadotropic hormone* activates the gonads; *prolactin* initiates and maintains milk production in new mothers;

MSH (melanophore-stimulating hormone) regulates the skin color and also has an influence on attentiveness to visual stimuli.

The posterior portion of the pituitary is connected by a stalk to the hypothalamus, which is closely associated with the pineal gland. The hormones of the posterior portion are actually manufactured in the hypothalamus, then transported for storage and secretion from the pituitary. These are *oxytocin* and *vasopressin*, both of which act on smooth muscle. Oxytocin acts on the uterus and the cells of the mammary glands during pregnancy, birth, and nursing. It has been linked with the "mothering instinct," initiating licking in animals and affectionate cuddling in human mothers and fathers. Vasopressin acts on the arteries, controlling the rate at which water is reabsorbed into the body by the kidneys.

The hypothalamus regulates the activity of the pituitary with its own hormones, called *neurohumors*. These are of two types: (1) *releasing and inhibiting factors*, which stimulate the anterior portion of the pituitary to release or prevent the release of its hormones, and (2) *endorphins*. Each set of hormones has its own releasing and inhibiting factors. For example, the growth hormone inhibiting factor *somatostatin* inhibits the release of TSH. It also acts directly on the pancreas to inhibit the release of insulin and glucagon and the enzymes associated with digestion. So, through this hormone, the hypothalamus controls digestion and hunger. Nine different stimulating or releasing hormones have been isolated in the hypothalamus.

Endorphins are a class of morphine-like chemicals that stimulate the pyramidal cells in the brain's limbic system, creating a feeling of euphoria and inhibiting the experience of pain. Some say these hormones account for the "runner's high" and may explain how mystics can walk on beds of hot coals and sit on nails without flinching. Pain researchers are trying to find natural ways to stimulate the release of these chemicals, so that chronic pain sufferers can find relief. Biofeedback and deep relaxation therapy, electrical stimulation devices such as the transcutaneous electrical nerve stimulation (TENS) machines used by back pain patients, light-and-sound machines, and antidepressant medications such as amitriptyline all address this part of the brain, encouraging the release and utilization of endorphins.

The *pineal gland* is a small pinecone-shaped organ located at the very center of the head. The pineal is the ultimate regulator of all the endocrine functions. If the pituitary is the "bandmaster," the pineal is the "Grand Master." It is only a quarter-inch long and weighs only 100 milligrams.

There are two known hormones secreted by the pineal gland: *melatonin* and *vasotocin*. It produces only a few millionths of a gram of melatonin per day. Melatonin exerts control over the hypothalamus (which turns the pituitary on and off). Vasotocin synchronizes menstruation, pregnancy, birth, and breeding cycles in animals by releasing or delaying release of oxytocin through the hypothalamus and pituitary glands.

The pineal gland is the body's biological clock, telling the body when to be active, sleep, eat, etc. Light affects the pineal gland by turning off the secretion of melatonin. Without the influence of melatonin, the hypothalamus stimulates the pituitary to go to work, activating all the other glands.

At night the pineal gland produces melatonin, blocking the release of the hypothalamus's releasing factors. Thus, the body's external activities are turned off.

Melatonin has been shown to calm the mind and prevent the brain from interpreting stressful stimuli in a way that overstimulates the adrenals. Yoga science has mentioned a "nectar" secreted at the top of the head during meditation, which creates a feeling of blissful ecstacy. This "nectar" may be melatonin. If so, meditation stimulates the production of melatonin.

Many people are unaware that the main purpose of yoga is to massage and systematically pressurize various glands. The purpose of a particular pose may be to address a certain physical condition such as constipation, an emotional condition such as anxiety, or a mental condition such as difficulty with concentration. But the overall goal is one of balance and harmony so that spiritual energy can be accessed.

## THE PSYCHOSPIRITUAL BENEFITS OF YOGA POSTURES

Yoga postures were invented as a means to help spiritual seekers attune their bodies to the growing capacity of the mind for expansion. You will notice, if you try to meditate or still your mind, that in the beginning your body rebels. Aches and pains, itches and twitches constantly interrupt your concentration and make spiritual bliss seemingly beyond attainment. Sometimes, if the mind is very strong but the body is weak, illness will prevent further meditation. We cannot ignore our bodies in an effort to expand and control the mind; they are intimately connected.

A daily practice of yoga postures makes the body fit for meditation and concentration by stretching and relaxing the muscles and ligaments, straightening the spine, oxygenating the blood, and balancing the secretions of the endocrine system. In this way, we work *with* our bodies, *through* our bodies to reach deeper states of awareness, rather than ignoring or escaping the body — the precious "container" of our deepest Self.

*Processes that help people release resentment, express negative feelings, and forgive past wrongs (whether real or imagined) may well be a major part of the preventive medicine of the future.*

— Carl Simonton, M.D., *Getting Well Again*

There are thousands of yoga postures. Out of these, only around forty are truly effective for normal people, and only a few are necessary for the individual. You need not contort yourself into a pretzel to be a practicing yogi! The postures given here are especially helpful for women and can be done by anyone. Because of their profound impact on the endocrine system, more advanced postures should preferably be prescribed by a qualified teacher who can analyze your constitution; your level of development; your physical, mental, and spiritual needs. If you have any specific problems, be sure to tell your teacher about them.

## RULES FOR YOGA POSTURES
• after bathing
• before eating
• in a clean, quiet, draft-free place
• in loose, nonbinding clothing
• not during menstruation or after the third month of pregnancy

## BREATHING

In order to be cleansed of dust and bacteria, air should be drawn in through the nose. The mucous membranes filter it and the antibacterial properties of their secretions kill many germs. In addition, the air is gradually warmed to body temperature by the longer route through the nasal passages. In yoga, long, slow, deep exhalation is emphasized, to remove stagnant air from the lungs and to get the most vital energy from the atmosphere. Slow, regulated breathing results in less work for the heart, lower blood pressure, relaxation of the body, quiet nerves, and a feeling of peace. When you breathe in, feel the air slowly fill your lungs completely, letting your stomach expand. With exhalation, squeeze the air out from the bottom up.

Each yoga posture requires a movement during inhalation, then a pause; a movement during exhalation, then another pause. Move slowly and pause fully, without tension. *Asana* means "a posture comfortably held." To strain or hold the postures in tension defeats their purpose.

## VITAL ENERGY AND THE BREATH

According to yoga philosophy, the energy that permeates the entire universe, animating everything from stars to amoebas to human beings, is *prana*, or vital energy. The Chinese call it *qi* (pronounced *"chee"*). It is the essence of life. It wraps our bodies and those of animals and plants in a subtle electromagnetic sheath; it emanates from us according to our state of mind and health. We breathe it in and we use it for everything we do.

This subtle energy has been discovered and rediscovered by sages and scientists throughout the ages. The Russian scientist Valentine Kirlian developed a method by which photographs of this energy field can be taken and studied. Russian physicians use Kirlian photography to detect the early stages of disease in the "bioplasma" long before it would ordinarily be discovered in the physical body.

Kirlian photographs of the hands of healers often show an intense, laser-like light emanating from the hand. In one experiment, E. Douglas Dean, of the Newark College of Engineering in New Jersey, took several sets of Kirlian photographs of psychic healer Ethel C. DeLoach. Comparing photographs of her fingers while she was at rest and while she was merely *thinking* about

*Air weaves the universe. Breath weaves human beings.*

— *the Upanishad, Atharva Veda*

79

healing, remarkable differences were found. When she thought about healing the flares and emanations from her fingertips were much larger and more intense. At one point she asked if he would like to see a green flare. Surprised at her apparent confidence about producing on demand, he set up the equipment. She closed her eyes and there, on the photograph, emerged a green flare of light.

At the UCLA Center for Health Sciences, Dr. Thelma Moss and her colleagues used Kirlian photography to observe healers and their patients. Each time, after a treatment, the corona of light around the healer's fingertip was diminished, while that of the patient was increased in brilliance and width. Volunteers with no experience in healing were not able to produce the same effect. It may be this powerful flow of prana, or vital energy, that heals, radiating from the electromagnetic field of the healer into the bioplasmic energy body of the patient, balancing and revitalizing the body through radiant energy.

People who have a "green thumb" may be describing the prana they are able to transfer to plants. In another series of experiments at UCLA, leaves were photographed after being freshly picked from the same plant. Then each leaf was mutilated and photographed again. This caused the emanations from the leaf to become much dimmer. A group of people with "green thumbs" — who seemed to have the ability to raise flourishing plants — were asked to hold their hands above the leaf. The newly photographed leaf showed an increased brightness in the bioplasmic emanations and remained brighter for many weeks longer than the untreated leaves. Conversely, people who claimed to have a "brown thumb" — meaning plants seemed to get sick and die under their care — were tested the same way. The light around the leaves virtually disappeared.

Kirlian photographs show intense changes in this energy field with fluctuations of emotions and thoughts. Photographs of the fingers of a calm, relaxed person show very small, bright emanations of blue-white light around the tip, while that of an angry person shows intense, chaotic red-orange flares streaming out of it.

This energy seems to be influenced by atmospheric changes as well, and especially by the electrically charged particles of the air. It is revitalized by negatively charged particles, near rushing water and dense foliage. A walk near a mountain waterfall causes us to breathe deeply, "drinking in" the air, which is redolent with the nourishing prana we need. Conversely, the bioplasmic energy body is fatigued and weakened by the positively charged particles that most proliferate under conditions of pollution, electrical wiring, heating and air conditioning, and dry, desert winds.

According to yoga, prana circulates throughout our systems via currents connecting the seven chakras with the glandular system. The Chinese medical science of acupuncture is based upon a knowledge of how to stimulate these subtle currents and balance them to create health. Interestingly, Kirlian photographs show energy flares in exactly the same points mentioned in acupuncture texts.

For thousands of years, practitioners of yoga have understood the relationship between the breath and the vital energy in and around our bodies. Deep, slow breathing generates and replenishes prana, as is confirmed by Kirlian experiments; the colored energy patterns around our bodies become much brighter when our lungs are filled with fresh, oxygenated air.

We absorb life-giving prana through our food and, even more importantly, through every breath we take. But during ordinary breathing, we

All of us know the fact that the speech of some persons penetrates to the heart of the hearers while the speech of another will bring no effect on the mind, though he speaks beautifully. In the former, the speech is charged with prana and in the latter it is merely intellectual.

—— Swami Vishnudevananada

One ingenious hypothesis was developed by Dr. William Tiller at Stanford University. Tiller was impressed with the apparent relationship of location and function between the chakras and the endocrine glands. He wondered how these so-called etheric organs might interact with the glands. Drawing from concepts used by electrical engineers, he suggested that this interaction could be analogous to a process of transduction. Imagine great energy streams flowing through space and passing through our bodies, unabsorbed and unnoticed. Tiller suggests that perhaps the chakras can be tuned in to couple with this power source and transduce some of its energy from the astral or etheric levels into the glands. One can think of the chakras and glands as electrical transformer loads that will deliver maximum power if they are balanced with respect to each other.

—— Jeffrey Mishlove, Ph.D.,
*The Roots of Consciousness*

82

extract little of the vital prana from the air, and, working and living in environments of pollution, cigarette smoke, stale air, computers, and electrical currents, not much of what we breathe actually revitalizes our bioplasmic energy. Practicing systematic deep breathing, as is important in the practice of yoga postures, provides an entirely different kind of nourishment to our physical and energetic bodies. Concentrated breathing stores vital energy in the chakras, oxygenates the blood, and refreshes the mind.

## How to Breathe during Warm-Ups, Yoga Postures, and Deep Relaxation

Through the breath we cleanse the lungs, the blood, and the tissues of our bodies. We revitalize the brain and nervous system, and we can calm or agitate our thoughts. When we master the breath, we master the mind.

Ideally, each breath is like an ocean wave, swelling and receding again and again in perfect rhythm. Yoga practice affords us the time to concentrate on this vital flow of nourishing air into and out of our bodies. The postures require this balance and utilize the important space between breaths to concentrate vital energy in the areas we need it most. You may wish to visualize a slow, rolling ocean wave as you teach yourself to breathe completely and effortlessly.

## Training the Body to "Breathe Itself"

Most people use only one-ninth of their body's full capacity for normal breathing. We breathe shallowly and inefficiently, and the result is chronic tension and fatigue. If we know how our lungs are *supposed* to work, we can begin to use our yoga session to train our bodies to breathe correctly and fully utilize all the wonderful prana available to us.

The trunk of the body consists of the thoracic cavity (the chest) and the abdominal cavity (the stomach). The lungs are suspended in the thoracic cavity, like bellows in a cage. The diaphragm is a thick muscle on the floor of the thoracic cavity. As the diaphragm descends and flattens (or contracts), air rushes into the lungs and the stomach rises. As air is expelled, the diaphragm rises and expands, squeezing the air out of the lungs. In yoga, we concentrate on the diaphragm, allowing our stomachs to rise as we breathe in and fall as we breathe out.

Use your first few yoga practice sessions to learn this diaphragmatic breathing. Eventually, your body will naturally breathe this way during your yoga practice, and you may find yourself naturally breathing deeply and fully at other times as well. Try it when you are tired, nervous, or for any reason you need to slow down.

## HOW TO BREATHE

(1) Relax on your back with your eyes closed. Place a pillow under your knees if you feel any strain on your lower back.

(2) Imagine your lungs filling in a wave-like fashion as you breathe in through your nose. The air slowly fills the top, then the middle, then the bottom of your lungs as your stomach gently rises. Hold for a fraction of a second, and feel what it is like for your lungs to be completely filled with fresh air.

(3) Now allow the air to leave slowly, through your nostrils. The wave recedes, and air is gently squeezed out from the bottom to the top, until no more air is left. Hold again, for a fraction of a second, and notice what it is

Thought commences and corresponds with vibration. When someone entertains a long thought, he draws a long breath; when he thinks quickly, his breath vibrates with rapid alternation; when the tempest of anger shakes his mind, his breath is tumultuous; when his soul is deep and tranquil, so is his respiration. But let him make trial of the contrary: let him endeavor to think in long stretches, at the same time that he breathes in fits, and he will find that it is impossible.

—— Emmanuel Swendenborg

like. On the next breath, allow your body to pull the air in slowly, and then slowly release it.

(4) Practice this breathing several times. If you become tense or feel dizzy or awkward, relax, breathe normally for a few minutes, and then try again. Gradually, it will begin to feel more natural, and you will need less concentration to carry the air in and out. You may need several sessions of practice to achieve this natural quality.

(5) When deep breathing feels more natural and your body is "breathing itself," begin to concentrate your mind on the place where the air meets your nostrils as it enters and leaves your body. Keeping the face and body relaxed and at ease, observe the air entering and leaving your body.

(6) When you have mastered this deep breathing, try counting the in-breath and out-breath. Start with a four-count (four counts breathing in, four counts breathing out). Adding a maximum of one count per day, gradually work up to an eight-count. Continue practicing at whatever level your body needs until it is easily "breathing itself" for a full count of eight on the in-breath and eight on the out-breath.

## RELAXATION

The art of deep relaxation has been practiced by yogis since ancient times, and instinctively by animals and babies. If you can truly relax for five to ten minutes, twice a day, you'll find your need for sleep decreased by as much as two hours. Complete rest refreshes and revitalizes the body in a very short period of time. The stresses of modern life drain your vitality and use up all the energy stored in your body. Experiments have shown that deep relaxation enhances learning and creativity.

In fact, many of the world's great discoveries were made in a state of total relaxation. For example, Charles Darwin, after years of gathering scientific data, suddenly "realized" his theory of evolution while taking a carriage ride in the country. Einstein developed the theory of relativity after spending an afternoon relaxing on a hillside. He let his imagination drift and found himself riding a sunbeam on a journey through the universe; eventually his drifting took him outside the realm of his scientific training. Curious, he went back to his study and worked out a whole new mathematical theory to explain what his "imagination" had told him.

Periods of relaxation and play allow the right hemisphere of the brain, the part that handles music, color, complex memory, images, and holistic thinking to function more fully and to integrate with the left hemisphere. Integrated hemispheric functioning helps us to think, act, and communicate more creatively.

The deep relaxation pose at the end of your yoga session is very important. In this pose, the mind's attention is gradually withdrawn from the body and absorbed in subtle consciousness. Your body and mind together attain a blissful repose. If you want to be energized by your yoga session, do a short (five minutes) relaxation pose at the end. If your prefer to be calmed and relaxed, do a short relaxation pose between each posture, and longer one (ten to fifteen minutes) at the end.

## GET READY FOR YOUR YOGA PRACTICE

There are several general guidelines to follow that will enhance your yoga practice and its effect on your body and mind.

(1) *Find your "best time" for your practice.* Yoga practitioners through the ages have suggested the best times for practice, and these are borne out by scientific studies of human cycles. Researchers have discovered what they call "ultradian rhythms," cycles of rest and activity that synchronize our bodily processes. Ultradian means "outside the limits of the day," and signifies short periods in which we naturally need to withdraw and rest. These cycles happen approximately every 90 to 100 minutes. At that time our thinking gets a little fuzzy, we may find ourselves yawning, gazing out the window, leafing through a magazine, or asking someone to repeat what they just said to us. We may wander to the coffeepot, thinking we need a boost, when actually what we need is to withdraw, relax, rest, and allow our minds to settle. During this time we naturally become ruminative, imaginative, and physically more quiet. If we can use this time for deep relaxation, yoga and/or meditation, we find that energy and clarity return. The synchronization of our brain's left and right hemispheres, our glandular "clock," our respiration and heartbeat, all bring us back to a state of readiness and activity. Fighting the "down time" makes us irritable and prolongs the feeling of tiredness, as the body struggles against the mind, each pulling in opposite directions.

Self-observation and experimentation will reveal your own ultradian rhythms, and you can try to synchronize your yoga session with the inward-turning, rest time of the cycle. You may wake up in this state if you are awakened by an alarm clock. If so, you can shower and do your practice right away.

If you wake up naturally, you probably awaken in an active state, and it may be an hour or so before you naturally wind down. If you practice in the evening, you may wish to observe yourself for a few days to see if there is a natural inward-turning time when you can schedule your practice.

Yoga practitioners advise the times around sunrise and sunset, well before eating a meal, as the best time for yoga and meditation practice. The science of biometeorology (the study of natural forces on human and animal life) tells us that the sun has a tremendous impact upon the lives of plants, animals, and human beings. Even our blood chemistry changes with the rising and setting of the sun! Therefore, there may be a chemical basis for the thousands of years of belief, in every spiritual tradition, that to meditate and pray at sunrise and sunset is somehow more effective, more auspicious.

Begin by scheduling your practice at the ideal times: morning and/or evening, before eating, near sunrise or sunset. Experiment with what feels right to you rather than following a strict routine. Eventually, you will find a good compromise and can settle into a comfortable rhythm with your practice.

(2) *Bathe*. Yoga may be practiced after your morning or evening shower. Alternatively, you may wish to perform a "half-bath," as yoga practitioners have done for centuries. A half-bath cools the body, relaxes the heart and nerves, and calms and clears the mind. Splashing cool water on the face automatically slows and regulates the heartbeat, activating the "diving reflex." This reflex is a vestige of our aquatic ancestors, whose nervous systems were designed to redirect the body's energies inward when diving into water. To perform a half-bath, use cool to lukewarm water in the following manner:

(a) Pour water over the genital area.

(b) Pour water over the legs from the knees down.

(c) Pour water over the arms from the elbows down.

(d) Splash water over the face, with eyes open, several times.

(e) Wash out your mouth.

(f) With a washcloth, cool the ears and behind the ears.

(g) With a washcloth, cool the back of the neck.

(3) *Practice in fresh air, away from drafts.* Yoga postures should be practiced indoors, out of direct sunlight and drafts, on a carpet or mat that slightly cushions the body. Performing the postures will create some heat in the body, and this is not a good time to expose yourself to a chill.

(4) *Keep the left nostril open.* There are two psychospiritual channels for vital energy (*prana*; see "Vital Energy and the Breath," p. 79), called *nadiis*, which weave through the chakras in the spinal column, ending in either nostril. When the breath is carried predominantly through the left nostril, the prana flows through the channel that keeps the body cool and the mind quiet but alert, and deep relaxation, meditation, and concentration are much easier to achieve.

How to clear your left nostril:

Lie down on your right side, resting your right ear against the inner side of your upper arm. Remain this way until the nostril clears.

Alternatively:

Sit cross-legged, with the left heel close to the body. Bend your right leg (upright), bringing the heel toward the body and the knee toward the chest. Lean the right armpit into the right knee and hold.

(5) *Do not practice yoga postures during menstruation.* To avoid causing excessive bleeding or cessation of menses, practice only the slow, easy warm-up stretches and deep relaxation pose (p. 106).

## WARMING UP

While yoga postures are vastly different from aerobic exercises, it is just as important to warm up the body before beginning the actual postures. In this chapter, we have learned the importance of breathing properly and how to do it, and we will experience several warm-up stretches, from which we can later choose our favorites for daily practice.

### FINDING CENTER

Begin your practice by settling into your body and finding your "center" — the place that keeps you in balance, physically and spiritually, and from which your energy arises. This is an important part of your yoga session and should not be overlooked; it prepares your mind to turn inward, and prepares your bodily structure to open to the postures that will follow. Ritualizing this part of your practice can provide a structure for your practice; you may wish to light a candle, or salute the four directions, or say a prayer before you begin. Starting this way creates a "border" between your regular day and your practice; when you step across the border, you are in sacred space — safe, comfortable, and completely relaxed, focused on yourself and the nurturing of your body, mind, and spirit.

## BODY LEVEL

Like the tool carpenters use to level a board, this exercise will help you find the "perfect center" of balance for your body.

(1) Stand erect, feet shoulder-width apart, arms at sides. Slowly begin to rock back and forth on the balls of your feet. Become aware of the exact point at which you feel perfectly "centered." Feel your energy connecting with that of the Earth through the soles of your feet.

(2) Now allow your body to lean to the right and the left, as far as you comfortably can without bending. Continue back and forth, until, finally, you settle at exact center. Close your eyes and feel this place.

(3) Now swing your body around in a circle, spiraling outward in bigger circles, and then gradually spiraling inward to center. Repeat, going in the opposite direction.

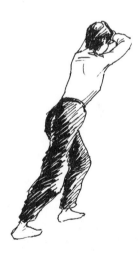

## STRETCHES

Start with some simple warm-up stretches. In the beginning, if you have difficulty doing any of the yoga postures, do these stretches instead. Slowly, as you become more flexible, you will be able to cut down on time spent on the warm-ups. These stretches can be incorporated into your day if your body is unaccustomed to sitting for meditation; they will limber the legs, back, and knees. They can be done during menstruation and pregnancy, when yoga postures are prohibited. Remember to breathe deeply and relax as you stretch — no bouncing, no forcing!

### (1) Calf Stretch

Facing a wall, stand a little distance away and lean your forearms on the wall with your hands crossed; lean forehead against your hands. Bend one knee and extend the other leg behind, both feet pointed straight ahead. Slowly move hips forward, keeping feet flat, until you feel a slight stretch in the calf muscles of the extended leg. Hold gently for a count of ten. Your body should be relaxed; don't overstretch. Alternate.

### (2) Quadriceps and Knee Stretch
Keeping one hand on the wall for support, reach behind and grasp the opposite foot. Hold gently for a count of twenty. Alternate.

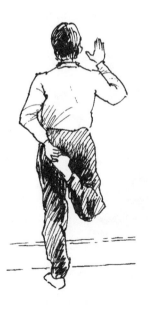

### (3) Groin Stretch
Sit on the floor with feet together, hands on your feet, and heels a comfortable distance from your body. Gently pull upper body forward, keeping your back erect, until you feel a stretch. Hold for a count of twenty. Relax arms, shoulders, feet.

### (4) Hamstrings Stretch

Straighten one leg, keeping the other leg bent with the sole of the foot facing the inside of the extended leg. Keep the extended leg slightly bent. Now bend forward slightly, from the hips, with arms relaxed on the floor next to the extended leg, until you feel an easy stretch. Touch the top of the thigh of the extended leg; it should be soft and relaxed. Keep the foot of the extended leg upright, not turned out. Hold for a count of thirty. Alternate.

### (5) Upper Hamstrings and Hip Stretch

Hold your bent leg to you gently, like a baby, with the other leg extended. Gently pull leg toward you until you feel an easy stretch. Hold for a count of twenty. Alternate.

## (6) Arch Stretch

Sit on toes with hands on floor in front for balance. Gently stretch the arches of the feet. Hold for a count of ten.

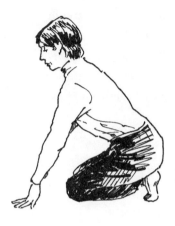

## (7) Arm Stretch

Hold one elbow with the other hand, over your head. Gently pull, relax, and hold for a count of twenty. Alternate.

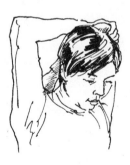

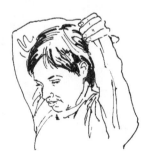

### (8) All-Over Stretch

Standing erect, touch palms together, arms extended forward.

Bring the arms slowly back to shoulder level. Then clasp hands behind back with arms extended straight down. Inhale deeply, pulling shoulders back. Exhale and bend forward, raising arms over head.

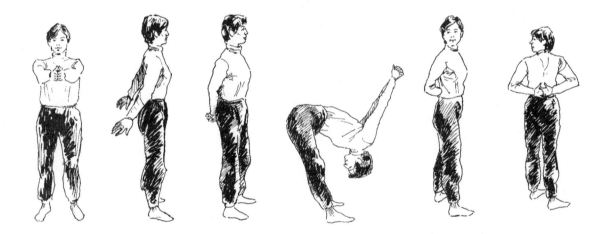

Return very slowly to original position, then slowly twist right and left. Repeat three times.

## (9) Back Stretch

Sit down and bring your knees up to your chest (ankles crossed), clasping them with both arms. Drop your head down to your knees and roll backwards on your spine. Roll forward and backwards several times.

 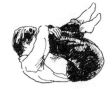 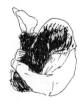

# YOGA POSTURES

**First Yoga Posture** (called Yogasana or Yogamudra)

Sit with your legs crossed and your back erect. With arms behind your back, grasp the left wrist with the right hand. Breathe out slowly as you bend forward to touch your forehead to the floor. If you can't reach the floor at first, just hold the posture at whatever point is comfortable. Hold for a count of eight. Breathe in slowly as you rise up again. Hold for a count of eight. Repeat

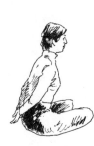

the entire cycle eight times. (Hint: If you haven't mastered the breathing yet, start with holding for a count of four and work your way up). When you hold the breath, do it in a relaxed way so that it is a quiet pause rather than a strain.

**Second Yoga Posture** (called Bhujaungasana or Cobra)
Lie down on your chest, with your palms on the floor near your head. Slowly raise up, looking toward the ceiling, breathing in. Keep the navel point on the floor. Hold for a count of eight. Return to the original position slowly, breathing out. Remember to keep your body relaxed as you hold the position. Repeat the entire cycle eight times.

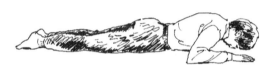 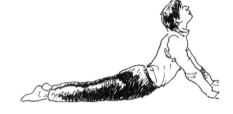

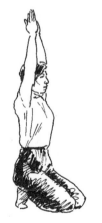

**Third Yoga Posture** (called Ardhakurmakasana or Diirgha Pranam)
Kneel upright, sitting on heels, supported by extended toes. Joining palms, extend your arms upward, keeping them close to your ears. Exhale and slowly bend forward, touching the floor with your forehead, trying to keep your hips in contact with your heels. Hold for a count of eight. Return to the original position, breathing in. Hold for a count of eight. Repeat the entire cycle eight times. If your arches are not flexible enough for this posture, you can do it with feet tucked under. Practice the arch stretch on page 93 until you can do this posture correctly.

## SELF-MASSAGE

A massage following yoga postures conserves the oily secretions of the sebaceous glands (keeping the skin soft and supple), stimulates the nervous system, relaxes the muscles, and enhances the circulation of blood and lymph. Lymph is a vital fluid that purifies the blood. It is not moved along lymphatic vessels by the pumping pressure of the heart; it moves solely by the action of the muscles. Massage thus greatly facilitates the flow of lymph. Special care should be taken to massage the areas of important lymph nodes: the neck, armpit, groin, and knee.

(1) Massage up the forehead, over the top of the head, and down the back of the head, with palms, three times.

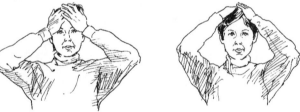

(2) With fingertips, massage out across the eyebrows three times.

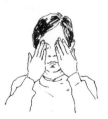

(3) With index fingers, press down in the crease between the top of the eye socket and the eyebrow. Pressure on this spot stimulates the vagus nerve to slow the heart, thus calming and relaxing the body and preparing it for the deep relaxation pose. Continue pressing with the fingers, moving them across the eyes, down the temples, in front of the ears, and around the back of the ears. Repeat three times.

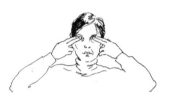 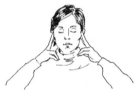 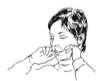

(4) Massage inside the ears.

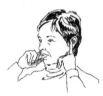

(5) With the outside edge of your palms, massage from the sides of your cheeks in toward the tip of the nose, three times.

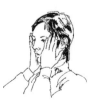

(6) With fingertips, massage under the eyes, and down the side of the face; then turn the hands sideways and massage the front of the neck. Then massage back across the sides of the neck and around the back, ending by massaging the back of the neck. Repeat three times.

 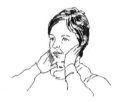

(7) Massage the upper lip three times.

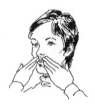

(8) Massage the chin area three times.

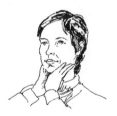

(9) With two thumbs, massage up inside the jaw starting under the chin and massaging outward toward the sides of the face, three times. This massages the lymph nodes and salivary glands.

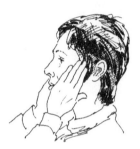

(10) With the palms pressed against the center of the neck, massage outward. This pressure on the center of the neck also affects the vagus nerve and lowers blood pressure. Repeat three times.

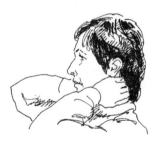

(11) Raise the arm and massage down the armpit with the fingers, three times. This massages the lymph nodes.

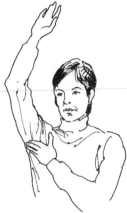

(12) Massage over the shoulder and down the upper arm. Then use a twisting motion to massage the forearm (follow direction of hair growth).

(13) Massage the back of the hand, the palm, and rotate around each finger. (Repeat with other hand.)

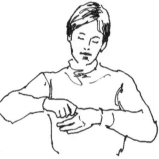

(14) Reaching up over the right shoulder with the right arm and behind the back with the left arm, bring your hands as close together as possible at the midback. Massage upward with the right hand and downward with the left. Reverse hands and repeat.

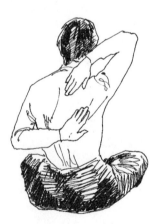

(15) Massage the chest, rubbing toward the heart.

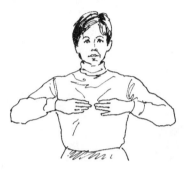

(16) Exhaling, place thumbs at sides of body and fingertips at the base of the ribcage. Massage out to the sides with fingertips, three times.

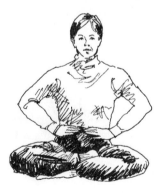

(17) Encircle both hands around the joint where the leg meets the trunk and massage this juncture. This massages lymph nodes in this area.

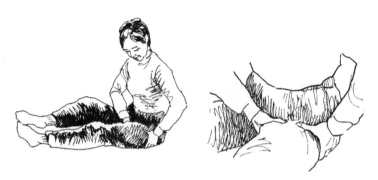

(18) Massage down the thigh, three times.

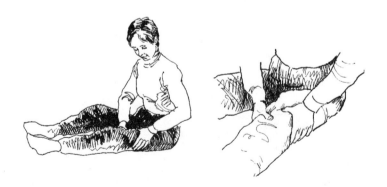

(19) Place right palm over kneecap and left hand under. Massage with a combined motion of the two hands. Then massage down the calf, following the direction of hair growth.

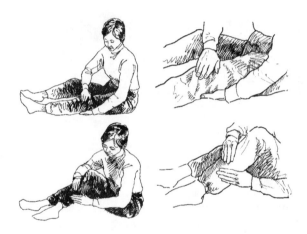

(20) Massage ankle with thumbs and fingertips.

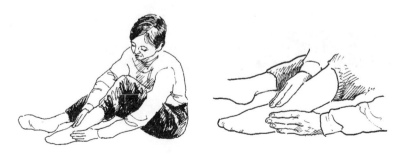

(21) Massage foot thoroughly with thumbs.

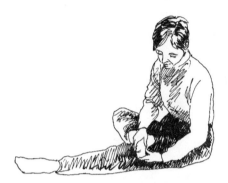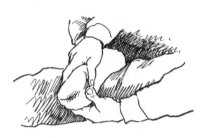

Now repeat (17) through (21) on the other leg.

**Final Yoga Posture** (called Shavasana or Deep Relaxation Pose)
Lie quietly on the back, palms up. Deeply relax each part of the body, starting with the toes. Practice for five to ten minutes.

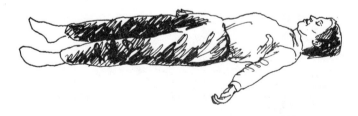

## ADDITIONAL POSTURES

The following two postures are for those who are strong and limber. If you are a beginner, wait until you have established a daily practice of warmups, performing the previous postures, and meditation before you add these to your routine. They work on the entire endocrine system, enhance circulation to the brain and thyroid gland, and stretch and align the spine. Do these postures after warmup stretches and before the self-massage.

**Shoulderstand** (called Sarvaungasana)

Lie down on your back. Gradually curl up, raising the body, supported by your hands. Slowly uncurl the legs until your body is in a straight line upward, chin in contact with the chest and feet relaxed. Look at your toes. After two minutes, slowly bring the legs back down into a curl, and lower yourself vertebra by vertebra onto the floor. Relax for at least one minute.

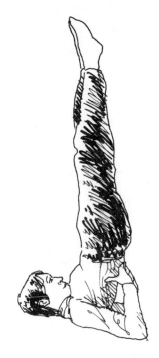

**Fish** (called Matsyamudra)

Lie down on your back and bring your feet up, one leg over the other, grasping each foot with a hand. Arch the back, with the top of the head as close to touching the floor as possible. Look at the tip of your nose, and rest your elbows on the floor. Hold, relaxing as much as possible, for one minute. Then stretch out and relax.

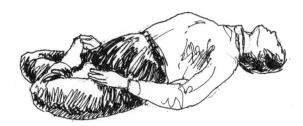

If you are unable to cross your legs on top, tuck them under you, crossed, holding each foot with the opposite hand.

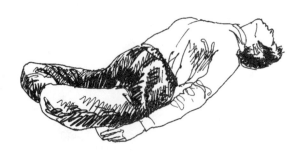

## EXERCISES

There are two categories of exercise: *low intensity*, such as isometrics, and *aerobic*, such as running. Yoga postures represent the first of these. Some aerobic exercise (rhythmic activity of the large muscle groups), in addition to yoga postures, will strengthen your cardiovascular system and increase your stamina. One exercise in yoga has this effect and also has the spiritual benefits of yoga postures. It is actually a "dancing" posture and is called *kaoshikii* (pronounced "cow-*shee*-kee"). It is the dance of mental expansion. A daily session that includes warm-ups, yoga postures, self-massage, relaxation, and kaoshikii will give you more all-around benefit than any other system of activity, plus the added benefit of directing both the body and mind's subtle energies toward your spiritual vision.

Like jogging or other aerobic exercise, kaoshikii should be adopted gradually. It may feel awkward at first, but soon you will feel its rhythm and pace and become comfortable with it. Kaoshikii can be done any time, but the best time is after your yoga postures, when your body is warmed up and relaxed and you are ready for the revitalization of this wonderful exercise.

Kaoshikii combines the benefits of meditation, yoga, and exercise. It has an *ideation* — a sequence of thoughts — that accompanies the movements. These thoughts, combined with the movements, help strengthen the mind. The heterolateral movements, which cross the midline of the body, help enhance left brain functions, while the homolateral movements, which extend the limbs, enhance the functioning of the right brain and bring the consciousness to a sense of surrender to the deeper Self.

### How to Do Kaoshikii

The dance consists of moving the upper body (with arms up and palms together, bending form the waist) to the right, to the center, left, center, forward to touch fingers to the floor, center, backward, and to the center again. As you do this, you are moving your feet in rhythm: the right foot touches the floor behind the left foot, then stomps the floor, flat. The left foot touches the floor behind the right foot and stomps the floor, flat. The dance ends with each foot stomping flat and the body upright.

Repeat the entire cycle as many times as you can, starting with three and gradually increasing, adding another round each week. Kaoshikii is the dance of the spiritual warrior. It prepares you to face the world with strength and courage. Practice as shown in the illustrations until you feel comfortable with it. Then you can add the ideation.

(1) Ready: arms up, feet a comfortable distance apart. ("I seek a link to the Infinite.")
(2, 3, 4) Bend to the right, touching right then left foot to the back, alternating. ("I request its presence.")

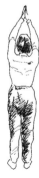 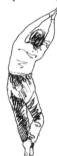 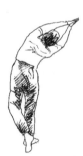 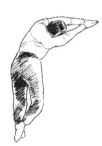

(5, 6) Continue touching right and left foot alternately behind. Bring arms up to "ready" position.

(7, 8, 9) Bend to the left, continuing the right-left step, toward left. ("I am a willing channel for infinite consciousness.")

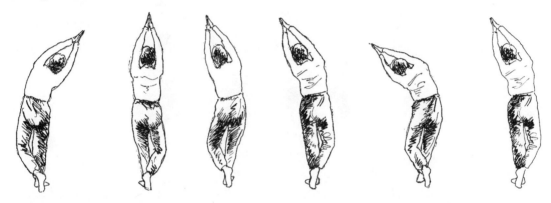

(10, 11) Continue right-left step, bring arms up to "ready" position.

(12) As right foot touches behind, arms are brought down in front.

(13) As left foot touches behind, fingertips touch floor. ("I surrender to my higher self.")

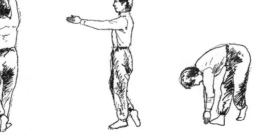

(14) "Ready" position with right foot touching behind.

(15, 16) Continue left-right step, leaning upper body backward. ("I am ready to face all obstacles.")

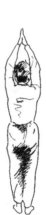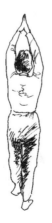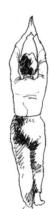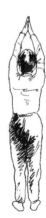

(17) "Ready" position with left foot touching behind.

(18, 19, 20, 21) "Ready" position; stomp the floor with each foot. ("I repeat the cosmic rhythm.")

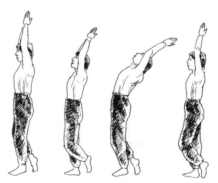

## BEAUTY SECRETS OF THE YOGIS

Everyone wants to be beautiful. Most people realize that beauty and attractiveness are essentially inner qualities, not merely related to our physical appearance. If you possess inner beauty you don't have to do much to enhance it. However, a few habits cultivated by yoga practitioners will help your natural beauty shine through and will contribute to the all-around health of body and mind. Cleanliness is truly "next to Godliness." Keeping the body clean is the yogi's most important health and beauty secret.

### SKIN

Take a full bath or shower once every day, using natural castile soaps and scrubbing all over with an abrasive sponge such as a loofa to remove dead cells and enhance circulation to the outer layers of the skin. Finish your bath with a cool rinse, and while your skin is still damp, use a natural lotion or cream to remoisturize.

### MOUTH AND NOSE

At least twice a day use a tongue cleaner or spoon to clean accumulations from the tongue. Especially in the morning, after sleep, after fasting, and when you are ill, a film from the digestive process builds up. Cleaning the tongue virtually eliminates the need for using a mouthwash, because along with a good brushing of the teeth, it gets rid of the bacteria that can cause breath odor.

It is also helpful to clean the nasal passages, especially when there is any blockage of mucous in the nose and throat. Here's how: Add about 1/2 teaspoon of salt to a small bowl of warm water. Bend over, placing your nose into the water, and gently pull some water through your nose. Spit it out, and blow your nose. The salt in the water acts as a germicide and also makes the process comfortable for tender mucous membranes.

## HAIR

Coconut oil is an inexpensive and natural conditioner for the hair. Once a week or so, comb some coconut oil through your hair and, if possible, take a steam bath (hot steam will help it penetrate). Leave it on overnight, then wash your hair in the morning. A few tiny drops of coconut oil combed through pubic and armpit hair once a day keep these areas cool and clean and act as a natural deodorant. Pouring cool water over the genital area after urinating also helps keep this area cool, clean, and odor-free.

## A NOTE ON DIET

Our food certainly has an impact upon us, both physically and psychologically. A well-balanced diet of fresh foods will aid in your spiritual work. However, food is also intimately tied to lifelong habits and psychological needs. I don't want to turn you away from meditation by telling you how to eat. Start meditating today. You don't need to change your life otherwise; meditation will bring to you intuitively the changes that will help you on your path toward self-realization. If you are interested in dietary changes that might enhance your spiritual practices, the recommended reading will give you a good start.

If you are having trouble concentrating in your meditation or if your body is generating a lot of heat during meditation, try eliminating some or all of the following foods: meat, fish, onions, garlic, eggs, mushrooms.

Recommended Reading:

*The Vegetarian Alternative* edited by Vimala McClure

*The Vegetarian Lunchbasket* by Linda Haynes

*Vegetarian Food for All* by Annabel Perkins

# Chapter Five
## Meditation

*It is not only for an exterior show or ostentation*
*that our soul must play her part, but inwardly*
*within ourselves, where no eyes shine but ours.*

— Montaigne

## COMPONENTS OF MEDITATION

Tantric meditation is taught in several components, each having a specific impact upon your mental and spiritual being, each helping you to gain access to the deeper layers of mind and to reach oneness with infinite consciousness. You receive these instructions when both you and your teacher feel you are ready for them.

### THE GURU

The Guru is that which leads to the goal. According to Tantra the only Guru is Brahma, the consciousness within us. But sometimes some external help and guidance is needed, and the student seeks a teacher. *Guru* means "dispeller of darkness." Having mastered the path, the Guru can provide many insights, show the pitfalls, and give instruction and correction that can speed your development.

It is through meditation that an internal relationship with the Guru is first established. Most people, when they meet their Guru in person, realize that a relationship already exists that has been wrought through their meditation. This relationship is very deep and very subtle, and, for the most part, it cannot be described. The Guru cannot be sought after. An old yogic saying is, "When the student is ready, the teacher appears." In the depth and stillness of meditation, at the time that is right for you, the Guru will make himself or herself known. You do not need a teacher to make a lot of progress in meditation. Trust that if and when you do need some external guidance, you will be led to the appropriate source.

## MANTRA

A *mantra* is a collection of sound vibrations uttered silently in the mind as a part of the meditation process. As was discussed earlier, the mind must always have some sort of object to which it attaches itself. You use this characteristic of mind in meditation by giving it an infinite object to dwell upon, to identify with, and ultimately to become. The mantra is your tool in this process. The sound of the mantra helps to still the mind, and contemplating its meaning helps to expand the scope of the mind infinitely.

The vibrational wavelength of the mantra is very subtle and so has the capacity to still the mind and bring it into harmony with the infinite. This is achieved through rhythmic sound vibration and repetition. The mantra is the linking vibration between the cosmic rhythm and the individual rhythm.

Another important quality of the mantra is *ideation*. Ideation, in its simplest sense, is to associate meaning with the mantra as it is repeated in the mind during meditation. It is not so much "thinking about" the meaning of the mantra as it is uniting thought and feeling and directing them toward identification with the infinite, at the same time that you are fully attending to the sound vibration of the mantra itself. These actions are not separate, as would be saying the mantra and then thinking its meaning or translation.

In the beginning you may simply associate the peaceful feeling of sitting by a mountain stream with the mantra; as your meditation progresses your perception of the goal expands and limited concepts fall away. Ideation is perhaps the most important aspect of the process; the feeling with which you approach your meditation can greatly help or hinder it. Halfhearted or mechanical repetition of the mantra will get you nowhere, but if your meditation is saturated with love you will be successful.

Once there was a great yogi walking along the shore of a river. He heard a woman, obviously advanced in yoga, chanting a mantra incorrectly. He thought it was his duty to correct this unfortunate person, so he crossed the river in his boat to the place where the woman was meditating. He corrected her, and she thanked him. He felt very self-satisfied; after all, it is said that someone who could repeat the sacred mantras correctly could even walk on water. As he was thinking this, he suddenly saw a strange sight. From across the river, the woman was coming toward him, walking on the surface of the water, bathed in light.

"My brother," she said when she was close enough, "I am sorry to bother you, but I must ask you again the proper way to repeat the mantra; I can't seem to remember it."

This story illustrates the significance of an intuitive approach. This isn't to say that correctness in form is not important. Though the most important aspect of a piece of music may be the feeling it evokes, the sound of the music is essential for the conveyance of that feeling. To express the highest intentions of the composer, every musician in the orchestra must be in perfect attunement with every note of music she plays. So, though ideation may be the most important aspect of the use of the mantra, its pulsative and incantative qualities are equally indispensable. Later in this chapter we will learn how to meditate using a universal mantra.

## LIVING MEDITATION

As you build a rich inner life through regular meditation, as your powers of concentration and visualization increase, so does your ability to actualize yourself in the outer world. Your mind becomes a very powerful tool. Earlier we discussed the mind's power to create, to impose, and to react, and the resultant samskaras. *Living Meditation* — the practice of consciously seeing the Supreme in all beings and circumstances — keeps the mind in harmony with the universe and reminds you of the oneness of all things. Keeping a vibrational rhythm and ideation of unity in the mind enables you to avoid creating further binding reactions by your thoughts and actions. It gives you a source of real power from which to act — not the limited power of the personal ego but the limitless source of universal power, which enables you to think clearly, act decisively, and give selflessly. This can be done in many ways. I suggest you begin by choosing a task you don't enjoy. Bring a conscious awareness of every moment to the task. For example, I used to really hate doing laundry. By applying the principle of Living Meditation, I was able to become present for it, to gradually stop repeating, "I hate this," over and over in my mind, and finally learn to enjoy and even look forward to it.

I began by bringing awareness to every physical aspect of the process: the weight of the basket, the sound of the water running, the feel of the clothes, the colors. I'd watch the detergent as I poured it in, noting its color, its texture, and scent — the feel of the lid as I shut it. I would meditate while the washing machine worked its magic. My gratitude went out to those who contributed to its invention as I let my mind flow to the rhythmic sounds it produced. Because of the technology, I was relieved of the hardship of pounding my clothing on a rock somewhere, and was given the luxury of a few moments to meditate.

I continued my awareness as I removed the clothes from the machine and placed them in the dryer, noting their fresh scent and the feeling of the damp fabric in my arms. Removing the clothes from the dryer became a much-anticipated joy: the lovely warmth and fresh, clean smell, the soft and varied fabrics, the feeling of accomplishment as I lovingly folded each garment, taking the opportunity to send love to its wearer (including myself!).

I highly recommend you try this practice. You will find, after a while, that not only do you begin to enjoy the task you previously dreaded, but the experience of spirituality in something usually considered mundane will begin to overflow into all the mundane tasks of daily life, and you will begin experiencing the inner harmony of the true Tantric.

Another component of Living Meditation is related to this consciousness of unity, but specifies an even deeper awareness — a surrender of the limitations of the ego to the limitless divinity within. It is called "Guru Puja" (offering to the Guru) and is performed following meditation. Through visualization you offer all past, present, and future thoughts and actions — all the "colors of the mind" — to the Guru (which is infinite consciousness, your "higher self").

When you have finished your meditation, kneel comfortably, with hands cupped together in front of you, eyes closed. Imagine all the experiences of your past, good and bad, becoming flowers of many colors, filling your hands. When they are filled, offer these imaginary flowers at the feet of your Higher Self, placing them on the floor in front of you. Again, imagine everything you are experiencing right now filling your hands with various colored flowers, and offer them. Finally, imagine your future, all the things you hope and fear, becoming flowers of all varieties and colors, filling your cupped hands. Offer these in complete surrender.

Through the practice of Guru Puja, you release all your attachments and qualities, both positive and negative, back to their source. It is an act of clearing the mind, of flinging open all the doors and windows in your temple of consciousness to let a fresh breeze flow through and all the built-up mustiness dissipate.

By letting go again and again, you begin to feel and realize that nothing is truly outside of you. You can never be truly alone. For example, you have a deep attachment to your child. The love you feel for her is a positive and dynamic force and is essential to her growth and well-being. But the kind of attachment that can make you overly fearful, dominating, protective, or clinging can be detrimental to both of you individually and to your relationship.

People often fear that by letting go internally, they may lose the object of their attachment. Actually, what you will find is a deepening, an enrichment of feeling, when the limits of a relationship are expanded by surrender of the ego's false sense of control. Guru Puja and Living Meditation help you to feel oneness and freedom from limitation.

## WHERE, WHEN, AND HOW?

I recommend you spend some time creating a routine of spiritual practice in your life. With the help of this book, you can do plenty of work before you take the step of searching for a teacher, if you choose to do so. Make a space, somewhere in your house, for your daily practices. It should be a quiet place, if possible, where people won't disturb you. It will become a sacred place for you; a place of peace and power. It can be a whole room, or just a corner. Place things there that focus your spirit and that make you feel good: a nice rug, a small table where you can place a candle or incense or some treasured items, a folded blanket on which to sit for meditation. Go to this special place every day — twice a day if possible — to nourish your body, mind, and spirit. People usually find the best times are early in the morning (an hour before breakfast) and/or in the evening. In the beginning, if you are unaccustomed to meditation and yoga, start easy. Reward yourself for consistent practice and increase gradually, if possible, from fifteen minutes of meditation to half an hour.

Cool your body first with a half bath (see p. 87) — splashing cool water over the lower legs, arms, and face. This refreshing yogic technique helps accelerate circulation while decreasing the workload of the heart; it energizes at the same time it relaxes the body. You may find that cooling off before meditation helps you concentrate and center yourself more easily as well.

Turn off the ringer on the phone and let friends and family know that during this time you do not wish to be disturbed. Close the door, close your eyes, and leave the ordinary world behind.

The short cold bath is more useful and desirable in changing the functions of the body than any other form of therapeutics.... It stimulates the thyroid to normal activity. It keeps the bone marrow functioning properly. It is an important prophylaxis against colds.... It should be utilized more frequently than it has been.

— Agatha Thrash, M.D.
and Calvin Thrash, M.D.,
*Home Remedies*

## HOW TO MEDITATE

Sit erect, cross-legged, on the floor if possible, with hands folded in your lap. Folding a blanket to support your "sitting bones" and tilting your pelvis forward can help align the spine properly. This position is best for meditation because it "locks" your energy in your body, enabling you to withdraw from the outer world. If it is uncomfortable for you to sit this way, find another position — preferably upright but relaxed.

Take a deep breath, filling your lungs completely with air. Hold for a moment, then slowly blow the air out, releasing tension with it. Repeat this process a few times, until you feel relaxed. Now imagine yourself in a special place, a place that makes you feel good. It could be near the ocean or in the mountains, anywhere. Imagine the air is full of *prana* — the vital energy of the cosmos — and you are breathing it in and out. Become one with all that is around you. Keep your attention gently on your breath, moving in and out. Let thoughts come and go without disturbing you; imagine your thoughts are birds, flying through the clear blue sky of your mind. They come, you are aware of them, and they fly away. Keep your attention gently on your breath. Now begin the ideation: as you breathe in, say silently to yourself, "All is . . ." and as you breathe out, say, "one." Repeat the phrase over and over as you allow your body to breathe itself.

Your mind will wander. Sometimes you may end your session having wandered so far you don't remember saying the phrase more than once. Release frustration with the breath, and just gently bring the attention back to the ideation. Have patience with your body and mind; they need time to become accustomed to this practice. After several weeks, you may add the mantra Babanam Kevalam (pronounced "*Bah*-bah-nahm *Kay*-vah-lahm") to your meditation. By now you will be accustomed to intoning its meaning, "All is One." You may repeat Babanam on the in-breath, Kevalam on the out-breath, ideating on the meaning as you do so.

## Suggested Schedule for Beginners

### Morning

(1) Upon rising, take a bath. If you find it helpful, sing or play some soothing music while you bathe, to get your mind into a meditative mood. Greet the new day, offering your gratitude and blessings to all those who have gone before, who have given so much to the world to make life easier for you (15 minutes).

(2) Sit in your special place; greet your inner self. Meditate for fifteen minutes. Some people find it helpful to set an alarm so that they aren't concerned with the time (15 minutes).

(3) Do warm-ups, yoga postures, self-massage, and the deep-relaxation pose (20 minutes).

(4) Do three rounds of kaoshikii (3 minutes).

### Evening

(1) Perform a half bath with cool water (5 minutes).

(2) Sing or listen to music as you stretch, relax, and prepare your mind and body for meditation (5 minutes).

(3) Meditate (15 minutes).

(4) Do warm-ups, yoga postures, self-massage, and deep relaxation pose (20 minutes).

(5) Do three rounds of kaoshikii (3 minutes).

You will be amazed at the changes this simple program will make. Soon you'll find yourself with more energy, vitality, and an increased awareness of your body's rhythms. Your concentration and alertness will be heightened. You'll sleep less and more deeply. You'll find a calmness and clarity within that helps guide your decisions and your relationships with others.

## On Self-Acceptance

People in Western cultures tend to become discouraged when they don't instantly achieve the results they want. Actually, we are not qualified to say whether we had a "good" meditation or a "bad" one. Every meditation is good, because an effort has been made to calm and control the mind. It is this consistent effort, every day, that forges your character and develops in you a deep inner strength that will guide you through all the peaks and valleys of your life. Accept yourself at every point along your spiritual path, acknowledge how far you've come; then take the next step.

## MENTAL AND EMOTIONAL WELL-BEING

When you begin a regular practice of meditation, your outward-focused energy will become balanced with an inward-turning awareness. At times you will encounter, within yourself or as a result of your circumstances, forces that set you off course and require more of your attention. These may be patterns created in childhood, as a result of negative experiences, or fears that have accompanied you from past lives into this one. Sometimes these psychological patterns can be so strong that they hinder your progress in meditation. Tantra recommends two ways of balancing the mind and emotions, through techniques using autosuggestion and those using "outer suggestion."

## Autosuggestion

The term autosuggestion means, simply, change motivated from within. As we have discussed, one very good form of autosuggestion is internal repetition of, and ideation upon, the mantra. Two other types of autosuggestion that work very well for the yoga practitioner are visualization and affirmation.

The specific techniques you use will depend upon your personality and what works best for you. First, analyze yourself; do you respond most to seeing, hearing, or feeling? One way to find out is to notice how you phrase things when speaking. Your verbal cues say a lot about you. People who are visually oriented say things like, "This is how I see it," "You should have seen that," "I see," "I can just picture him doing that," "Show me," "Look." People who are auditory respond this way: "Tell me about it," "I hear what you're saying," "Listen." Those who are more kinesthetic, or feeling-oriented say things like, "I feel you're wrong," "He's so touchy," "I lean toward that opinion, "I need to get a feel for it." For example, three friends describe a day at the beach:

Susan: "It was great! You should have seen the waves! The beach was so clean — pure white sand, and little shells everywhere. I found a beautiful pink one. The sun was so bright, and the sky so blue! Look, I brought a picture of it."

Margaret: "The waves crashed against the shore, and the gulls made such a racket! Then at sunset, everything became quiet and serene."

Ann: "Oh, and the feel of the warm water — it was like rocking in a big womb! The sand was so warm and squishy, and the air so clean and fresh."

Of course, we all use all of our senses to perceive and describe our experiences, but most people do express one more than the others; some people are dominant in two of these modes. In using the following techniques, you'll find that approaches that utilize your orientation will be the most effective. In fact, you can design any system to fit your needs. For example, a "visualization" exercise can include predominantly feeling-images or sound-images.

## VISUALIZATION

Many diseases have been arrested or cured by the patient's use of imagery. These techniques have been used with particular effectiveness by children, whose defenses and rigidity toward the free-flowing imagination are not yet developed. Meditation, by calming our minds and focusing on the expansive thought of the infinite, helps us revitalize that often dormant part of ourselves. Many of the practices you learn later on include the use of visualization of the chakras and energies of the psychic body.

The imagination is in the realm of the higher mind, where all knowledge resides. By using your conscious mind to direct images inward, you allow the unconscious to function in assisting the lower layers to heal the physical or psychic body. It is a means of getting your programming — those things you have absorbed or have been taught that may not be true — out of the way.

There are as many ways to visualize as there are people. A good way to do it is to write a script for your visualization, incorporating things that are meaningful to you in pleasing ways. Then make a tape of your script and play it to yourself at night before going to sleep or after your yoga postures, as you lie in the deep relaxation pose. Here is one example of a visualization you might use for healing:

## A HEALING VISUALIZATION

*Lying in a comfortable position, relax your entire body. Breathe in deeply, then out, several times. You will notice that with each inhalation you become more deeply relaxed, and with each exhalation tension melts away from your body. Starting with your toes and feet, focus your attention gently, and feel your muscles, your tendons, your bones, getting warm and heavy and completely relaxed. Move your attention up to your ankles, then your calves, knees, and thighs, gently focusing, feeling warmth and relaxation in each part of your body. Continue until you have inwardly spoken to every cell of your body, and you are completely, deeply, warmly, relaxed.*

*Now imagine yourself in a special place: a place that's just for you. It is exactly as you would like it to be, with everything you need available to you. Imagine it in every detail: how it looks, feels, smells. What colors are there? What textures? What objects? Now focus your attention on your body again, and allow it to tell you what it needs to heal. Wait patiently for the answer, each breath relaxing you more deeply.*

*Now imagine a beautiful light, a beautiful sound, or a beautiful feeling, surrounding and penetrating your body, sinking into your skin, your blood, every cell. This light, sound, or feeling is capable of healing you completely. It is drawn from the universal storehouse, where all things are known, and where perfection resides. It comes from a place where there is no disease, and it has the power to heal you completely. Feel its healing energy. Breathe it in, and* out. You can carry it with you, and if you need more, it will always be available to you.

When you wish, gradually return to the conscious world, comfortable in the knowledge that everything you need is already with you.

## AFFIRMATIONS

An affirmation is a positive statement. It is used to replace negative assumptions that can block your progress. The subconscious mind, being very absorbent, often takes as truth statements or past experiences that may not be helpful to you here and now. Your internal belief system can be based on these, and thus your own beliefs can undermine you, short-circuiting the new information that outdates these assumptions. For example, if someone is told again and again in childhood that she can't do math, it is very likely that she will grow up with this belief deeply entrenched in her mind. It becomes an imposed momentum. Every time she is faced with a mathematical problem, she will be uncomfortable, perhaps even panicky, and she will again hear that voice droning, "You can't do math."

A mantra is one kind of affirmation, though simple, positive statements are the most common form of affirmations. They give new information to your mind, countering old assumptions that you are limited, "only human," that perfection isn't possible. Affirmations are fun to use and can help you keep your mind in the open, positive state that is conducive to growth and success. To use them effectively, you'll want to find statements that ring true to you and that challenge a part of your beliefs you sincerely want to change. Obviously, parroting a statement that is too far from what you believe is possible will not help.

In an exercise to help identify and change false assumptions, we'll use the example of our friend, the mathematician — call her Sandra. Sandra would use two sheets of paper; the left one is for her affirmations, the right one for her subconscious responses. She writes "I love math, and I'm good at it," on the left-hand paper. Immediately, she'll probably hear an annoying voice — let's call it the "Inner Critic" — from her subconscious mind say something like, "Yeah, and I'm the Queen of England!" Sandra writes that down on the right-hand paper.

Again, she writes the affirmation on the left, and there's that voice again: "You can't do math!" She writes it down, and says something like, "Thank you for your input," to her Inner Critic. Then she writes her positive statement again. She continues to do this until the Inner Critic gives way. Perhaps after awhile, her Inner Critic will say something like, "Well, maybe you've improved over the years." Later she might concede, "I suppose it is possible." And finally, she'll agree, "Okay, so I was wrong. You can do math." Sandra tears up the list of negative responses and continues to write her affirmation every day for a few weeks. If she's really determined, she might draw it in big, colorful letters and post it on her refrigerator. She might record it on tape and play it to herself on the way to work. Then she can forget about it and enjoy being good at math for the first time in her life. If she's really motivated, she can begin taking math courses to sharpen her skill, confident that her subconscious mind will assist rather than hinder her.

This simple principle can be used in a wide variety of ways. You might want to identify obstacles in your meditation; perhaps they are assumptions rather than realities. Try to get to the bottom of whatever gets in your way; is it that you don't have time, or is some underlying fear the real reason you haven't set aside time for meditation? You can use visualizations and affirmations to help change your "self talk" when you feel stuck.

## MAKING YOUR OWN AFFIRMATIONS

Following this section I've included an example of an affirmation exercise you might use. I've filled in the "Clearing Response" side (that's our good old friend the Inner Critic) so that you can see what it might look like. Do five to ten sets in the first, second, and third person, once a day for a week. When your "Clearing Responses" have tapered off, make a cassette tape for yourself, repeating the affirmations in the first, second, and third person. Say the affirmation slowly, changing the feeling emphasis each time you say it; wait a few seconds before repeating it again.

If you have two tape players, you might try playing your affirmation tape along with a tape of music. Baroque classical music has been proven to be an aid in accelerated learning. Why? Because its heartbeat pace induces deep relaxation and breathing; when you are deeply relaxed and breathing freely, information is easily absorbed by the deeper layers of your mind. Vivaldi's "Four Seasons" or Pachelbel's "Canon in D" are perfect; adagio, larghetto, or largo movements from concertos by baroque composers usually have the sixty-beats-per-minute rhythm that is most conducive for this type of learning.

| Affirmation | Clearing Response |
| --- | --- |
| "I, (your name), enjoy meditating twice a day." | "It's so hard to sit there, and nothing happens anyway." |
| "I, (your name), enjoy meditating twice a day." | "I can't concentrate at all. I don't have time to do it right so I shouldn't do it at all." |

"I (your name), enjoy meditating twice a day."

My back hurts."

"You, (your name), enjoy meditating twice a day."

"I should have started a long time ago."

"You, (your name), enjoy meditating twice a day."

It is nice sometimes."

"You, (your name), enjoy meditating twice a day."

"I do sleep better when I meditate regularly."

"(Your name) enjoys meditating day."

It makes me feel good twice a about myself."

"(Your name) enjoys meditating twice a day."

"Who knows, maybe I'll have one of those peak experiences I've." heard about!"

"(Yor name) enjoys meditating twice a day."

"Yes I do!

Affirmations work best if they are short, simple, and phrased in the present tense; "I am strong and confident" is better than "I will be a strong and confident person." Also, phrase your affirmation in a positive way: "I am strong and confident," rather than "I am not weak."

## SAMPLE AFFIRMATIONS

"The more receptive I am, the more I receive."
"I am able to focus effortlessly on anything I choose."
"I have an infinite supply of energy and draw on it continuously."
"I speak only with good intention."

"I naturally enjoy and share my feelings."

"All that I give is given to me."

"I keep only thoughts that are supportive to me and others."

"Every negative thought automatically triggers three positive thoughts in my mind."

"I nurture and support myself."

"Each and every day I become more loving, more open, and more effective."

"I keep my agreements effortlessly."

"I am clear and straightforward in speech and action."

"All problems are opportunities to grow."

"I am infinite consciousness every moment."

"Every day, in every way, I am getting better and better."

## OUTER SUGGESTION

Outer suggestion consists of things and people outside of you that can help you achieve mental and emotional well-being. These include books, tapes, therapies, and the advice and instruction of a friend or teacher. When you find something in yourself that needs to change, you have a wealth of information and support available to you. Sometimes talking to a counselor or psychotherapist can help you sort things out and find solutions to problems.

When choosing someone with whom to share your personal journey, choose wisely. Interview several people recommended by others you trust. Don't settle for less than you deserve — someone who supports your spiritual journey and can communicate well with you. In Tantra, there are several types of outer suggestion to aid you in adjusting the subjective approach of meditation with the objective world. These include a code of ethics, a set of guiding supports and the comraderie of others in a spiritual community. The ethical precepts will be covered in Chapter Six.

## COMMUNITY

Humans are tribal by nature, and spiritually we are driven to find our place with others. You will find that it is much easier to continue your spiritual practices if you are able to meditate with other people regularly. Association with others, especially those who have been meditating longer, will have a positive effect upon your own meditation. If there is no ongoing group meditation in your area, you may want to form your own group, gathering together with the common goal of strengthening and caring for one another in the spirit of oneness.

Begin your group meditation with music. Singing, chanting, or listening to someone singing uplifting songs can help bring everyone into the frame of mind conducive to meditation. Simple songs or chants with a universal theme, such as "We are one in the spirit," or "We all come from God," work well to bring everyone together. The beauty of group meditation is in the powerful energy created by one focus on the infinite.

There is an ancient Sanskrit chant used by some groups for this purpose. Pick a low, comfortable musical tone and chant it all on that single note. You can chant the English words as well, if you wish. Under each Sanskrit line is a pronunciation guide:

*Samgacchadhvam, samvadadhvam*
sung gacha dwung sung wa dah dwung

*Samvomanamsi janatam*
sung wo manung see jah nah tum

*Devabhagam jatapurve*
day wah bah gum ja tah purr vay

*Samjanana upasate*
sung jah nah nah oopa sah tay

*Samaniva akuti*
sah mah nee wa akoo tee

*Samana hrdaya nivah*
sah mah nah hree dah yah neeva

*Samanamastu vomano*
sah mah nah mahs too woh mah no

*Jatavaha susahasati*
Jah tah wah ha soo sah ha sah tee

Translation:
Let us come together
Let us sing together
Let us come to know our minds together
Let us share like sages of the past
That all people may enjoy the universe.
Our hearts are as one heart
Our minds are as one mind
As we, to know one another, become one.

Recommended Reading:

*Beyond the Superconscious Mind* by Avtk. Ananda Mitra Ac.

*Woman Spirit: A Guide to Women's Wisdom* by Hallie Iglehart

*The Relaxation and Stress Reduction Workbook* by Martha Davis, Matthew McKay, and Beth Eshelman

*The Woman's Book of Spirit* by Sue Patton Thoele

# Chapter Six
# Tantra's Code of Ethics

*One falsehood spoils a thousand truths.*
— Ashanti proverb

The practice of Tantra yoga embraces every moment of our lives, and so our ethics — our guiding principles of conduct — are of course essential to reflect upon and study.

The way you conduct your outer life complements your meditation. With a balance of inner development and outer restraint, a sense of strength, of peace and clarity, stays with you all the time. Right conduct is the foundation of spiritual practice. Meditation without morality is useless; morality alone, though admirable, is not the goal of life. Because right behavior is often a struggle, the strength of mind afforded by regular meditation is a necessity. The guidelines below are thousands of years old, developed by the yogis as a way of bringing spiritual realization into a social context. They are not "commandments" but guides that must be deeply contemplated and rationally adjusted.

## ACTS OF INTEGRITY (YAMA)

### (1) SIMPLE KINDNESS — AHIMSA

The essence of the practice of Ahimsa (pronounced "ah-*heeng*-sah") in daily life is simple kindness; kindness to ourselves, kindness to others, and compassion when making social and political choices. The word *Ahimsa* means, literally, nonharm (*a*=no, *himsa*=harm); so this kindness includes refraining from inflicting harm upon other beings.

True Ahimsa must begin with an acknowledgment of the aggressor in us — the dark, ruthless side of ourselves as human beings. Stephen Levine, in *Healing into Life and Death*, speaks of "taking tea" with our dark side:

> Most people are basically kind and gentle but haven't yet cured themselves of the reactive, injurious quality of their anger. Few have taken tea with their outrage or confusion. Most try to push it away, causing it to explode unconsciously into a world already overflowing with violence and reactivity. Few, in order to cultivate the quality of harmlessness in their lives, have taken responsibility for their anger. To take responsibility for our anger means to relate to it instead of from it. To be responsible is to be able to respond instead of having to react.

We have many opportunities to explore our destructive side, to discover and acknowledge the parts of ourselves that are capable of atrocity. Parents know the powerful forces of love that go quite beyond the soft and gentle lullaby. Threaten to harm my child and I can easily take your life. So much for nonviolence.

But Ahimsa is not nonviolence. The natural order of the universe is violent; we cannot live one minute without taking a life. We must breathe and thus destroy millions of microbes, we must eat to survive, we must protect ourselves and others from harm, sometimes by doing harm to an aggressor. The spirit of Ahimsa is the effort to bring to consciousness our impulses to do harm, and to make choices that reduce the needless harm we do. It is a way of striving to be synchronous with that which is true human nature, which, in yoga's view, is compassionate.

Rather than a "commandment," Ahimsa must be chosen with care and understanding of the motivation, the implications, and consequences of one's behavior. This way of living requires constant attention, thought, and choice — for it means deeply feeling the things we do (or refrain from doing) for ourselves and others. We must choose what is congruent with our most honest understanding of each situation and its requirements of us.

Each of us has the capacity to harm and the capacity to bring understanding, forgiveness, and kindness to meet the demons of fear and rage, which cause us to harm ourselves and others. It is helpful to examine our harmful behavior with kindness toward ourselves, and then to consciously choose to practice behaviors that fuel our bodies and minds with positive energy, health, and integrity.

Ahimsa means, first of all, that we take care of ourselves; as much as possible, we do no harm to our bodies. We choose not to indulge in self-destructive recreational pursuits. We feed our bodies nutritious foods, bathe, exercise, and always try to see our bodies as beautiful, alive, and precious to us. We take time to nourish our bodies every day and special time to heal our bodies when they need healing. Aggression — that tense holding-on, which we can easily recall by imagining ourselves in a traffic jam on the way to an important appointment — sends waves of stressful impulses through our nervous systems, triggering the release of hormones that deplete our energy and undermine our immune systems. So practicing nonharm toward ourselves is more than simply refraining from harmful substances; it requires that we examine the stresses in our lives and learn how to reduce those that are

When kindness has left people even for a few moments, we become afraid of them as if their reason has left them.
—— Willa Cather

unnecessary and manage those that are unavoidable.

Emotionally, Ahimsa has to do with self-esteem, and with the way we turn our pain into weapons against ourselves and others. Practicing Ahimsa, we respect ourselves. Developing healthy self-respect requires that we heal the past. We try to bring to awareness experiences from childhood that injured us emotionally, experiences throughout our lives that have been harmful to us, and try to heal the damage and care for ourselves. It also means that we maintain self-respect within our relationships; that we learn how to say "no" when we need to, and how to gently but firmly let others know where our boundaries are.

Mentally, practicing Ahimsa means that we try to keep ourselves in situations that maintain our mental peace. It means we don't beat up on ourselves; neither do we constantly demand ourselves to accomplish things of which we are incapable.

Shame is a self-destructive mental addiction that can undermine our physical, mental, and emotional health and keep us from growing. It is the invisible "nitpicker" sitting on our shoulders, criticizing all that we do, berating us for what we haven't done, and telling us we're worthless. We may feel guilty or remorseful for something we did or did not do. We can choose to work through it with whomever we hurt and clean up the damage caused by our action or inaction. Behavior can be changed. But shame, which is often triggered by guilt, debilitates us. It is the feeling that we are intrinsically useless, irresponsible, ugly, bad, mean, etc.

Shame usually results from childhood abuse. When children are humiliated, blamed, degraded, criticized, disgraced, laughed at, teased, manipulated, deceived, betrayed, bullied, minimized, invalidated, and made the object of cruelty, sarcasm, and scorn, shame is the poison they internalize. While guilt involves actions that are forgivable and correctable, shame offers no hope — no way out. We can't do anything about it because it is us. Both guilt and shame are part of being human. However, sustaining an intimate relationship with shame uses up a tremendous amount of energy without accomplishing anything; it depletes us and eventually becomes resentment and anger, which are then acted out in our relationships.

In our relationships, Ahimsa requires that we do not intentionally hurt others — groups of people as well as individuals. We observe ourselves acting out anger, resentment, judgment, blaming and victimizing others. Where does this behavior come from? What triggers thoughts that make our hearts grow cold and cause us to think, speak, or act this way? With compassion toward the pain that lies beneath all of this rigidity, we can explore our thoughts and emotions and try to allow the issues that cause them to come into focus.

Anger itself is not against Ahimsa; rather, it is a feeling that calls for exploration. It is the acting out of anger, without mercy for ourselves and others, that violates the spirit of Ahimsa. When we don't have a healthy relationship to our negative states — our rage, our fear, our frustration — we suppress them or react in ways that hurt. This behavior creates more of the same — not the release we seek.

We can begin to explore our inner territory and discover what our anger conceals. Anger is like a scary mask. Behind it is a frightened, hurt child. We need to find that child and heal him or her; give her the safety and love she needs. The mask then becomes unnecessary and real communication can happen.

## AHIMSA IN PARENTING

Ahimsa in relationships also applies to our children. We can find ways to help nurture them, guide them, and allow them to develop healthy boundaries. And we can work on reducing behaviors such as criticism, blame, control, and ridicule.

Physical and verbal abuse clearly violate the spirit of nonharm in our families. But accepting kindness as a cardinal value does not mean we never feel angry. Parents experience moments when a child brings them to the edge of sanity, when physical or verbal abuse are distinct possibilities. In that moment can grow compassion for oneself and for others' pain — and true remorse, which makes us soften and brings us closer together. Out of that moment may also grow aversion, self-hatred, intolerance for others' struggles and shame, which hardens our hearts and pushes a wedge between us.

A parent who has adopted the value of Ahimsa is always working through feelings: exploring them and giving voice to them, finding ways to communicate them without causing damage, and learning how to guide a child with firm but supportive discipline. If we were hit and made the object of ridicule and sarcasm when we were children, if we were discounted and dismissed, it takes a conscious effort to choose other ways to discipline our own children, ways that may not be in our parenting repertoire. Acting out feelings impulsively won't work. We can find and practice ways to communicate with our children that let them know we respect them, and at the same time help them learn where our (and their) boundaries lie. Active listening, time-outs, negotiation, and choice-making are all skills that can be learned and used effectively to take the violence out of parental discipline.

Our children learn primarily by living in an environment that demonstrates how things are done. In short, they learn by our example. And more than ever, with the violence and materialism of a troubled world clamoring outside our doors, they need the security of core principles at home. Never before has the home been so important; never before has the example we give our children been so crucial as it is now.

## AHIMSA IN OUR SOCIAL AND POLITICAL CHOICES

Socially and politically, choices for Ahimsa can vary widely. As you begin to explore its depth and comprehensive applications to life, you will find more and more food for thought. Ahimsa alone could be the subject for an entire book. Here, I have attempted to confine the discussion to areas that are of particular concern to us as women and human beings in Western cultures.

## VEGETARIAN DIET

Most people who practice yoga gravitate toward a vegetarian diet not only for its nutritional benefits but because of a willingness to embrace this idea of nonharm. Naturally, if we start to think about the kinds of harm we inflict upon other beings, at some point we will think about the animals that are tortured and killed to feed us.

In selecting food, the spirit of Ahimsa is to choose food with comparatively less development of consciousness, judging by the capacity to express that consciousness. As my daughter says, "I don't eat things that could move off my plate by themselves if they were alive." The spirit of Ahimsa is to consider circumstances when making these decisions and to make them with reason and restraint.

In the United States today, over nine million creatures are slaughtered each day. We must ask ourselves if killing is a necessity we would undertake if each of us personally had to kill and dismember the animals we eat every day. Even if "humane slaughter" were possible, how would the act of killing itself change us, given the fact that we have no tribal culture, little daily kinship and interdependence with nature, no spiritual context within which killing for luxury can fit, and no necessity to do so?

Modern slaughterhouses and poultry farms — even dairies — are managed in such a way that the animals whose lives are taken are treated as things whose blood and breathing (so like ours) and screams of pain when tortured (so like ours) are denied, ignored, and silenced. How could it be otherwise? How could we, with consciousness and care, brutally take the lives of nine million creatures a day and stay sane?

## PASSIVE RESISTANCE

In India's epic *Mahabharata*, the Lord Krishna exhorts the Pandava brothers to take up arms against the Kaoravas, who have taken possession of the kingdom by force and are ruthlessly exploiting its people. A great battle ensues, wherein Krishna shows the warrior Arjuna that there are times when the only choice is to fight, and at those times the results must be surrendered to God. These stories have both internal and external significance. Sometimes the fight is the internal commitment to find our truest selves and follow our path, to hold on to our integrity and tell the truth. Sometimes the fight must take place in the world, with words or weapons.

Some people interpret Ahimsa as refusing to participate in war. Choices range from refraining from any violent struggle to evaluating its purpose and trying to decide where the harm lies. Sometimes the lesser of evils must be chosen. For example, the harm that is done by a ruthless dictatorship to millions of innocent people may be far worse than the harm that is inflicted by an armed struggle against it. So a choice to fight, while it cannot be characterized as nonviolent, may be upholding the cardinal value of Ahimsa.

Often Mahatma Gandhi's philosophy of Ahimsa is called nonviolence. But an examination of the history of India's struggle for independence reveals a cunning strategy of warfare, with the weapons of forbearance on one side and the weapons of brute force on the other. These weapons of forbearance are often more powerful than the weapons of brute force, and are but one of many difficult choices faced by leaders of a resistance movement. Hundreds of thousands of people were maimed and killed in India's struggle. It cannot be characterized as a nonviolent struggle, or even "passive" resistance. Rather, nonviolence was a carefully and actively selected tactic with full knowledge of its implications, just as if the resistors were to face police with Molotov cocktails. The people who followed Mahatma Gandhi subjected themselves (and were subjected by him) to violence in the extreme.

The "direct action" of ecology groups (which some call militant, some call nonviolent) — including blocking roads, sitting in small boats between whale and whaler, dismantling or disabling harmful equipment, and other "ecotage" actions to defend the environment — cannot be called nonviolent. However, these actions may be ethical under certain circumstances, when choices have been systematically eliminated. Any action that may endanger life or livelihood requires a great deal of thought and communication. Gandhi insisted that communication is the element which makes any "nonviolent" strategy work. Leaders must state the goals, announce intentions, and choose an action that most reduces the tendency toward harm or violence for all parties concerned. When an action is appropriate, it has great power, for it is in harmony with universal laws. Accepting Ahimsa, we work for justice without succumbing to judgment; we oppose without becoming locked into opposition.

## ABORTION

Ahimsa requires conscious thought. It is not something we can decide to follow, and then know what to do every day for the rest of our lives. During certain periods in our lives, we may evaluate it on a daily basis. There will be times when we are unable to find the right answer, and must finally choose a course and hope the results are what we want and can live with.

Practicing Ahimsa requires compassion both for the fetus, which is accepted as a living, incarnated being, and for the woman whose anguish no one else can feel. The decision to prevent birth is not an easy one, and must be made considering the suffering and pain of all within its circle.

Some Buddhists have a funeral ceremony for the fetus, which brings consciousness to miscarriage or abortion and allows the human need to acknowledge what has happened, to grieve and express remorse, and to send the soul of the departed on with respect and caring. Melody Ermachild wrote about one such ceremony:

As we speak, our intentions and our fates criss-cross, weaving the fabric of our complex women's lives. Outside of this room, judges on high courts make decisions while marchers hoist their picket signs. A bomb could explode in an abortion clinic. But we, as we sit, feel in our bodies what we know: She could be me, and I cannot judge her. . . .

    I gain a deeper understanding of the meaning of what it is to be "pro-choice." Choice is not control. . . . Choice is a dialogue with the being who may come to life through our body. We can do no more than to bring our awareness to this sacred conversation. Something is learned from every life and every death. Choice gives us freedom, and choice asks us to accept what we have done.

The spirit of Ahimsa is compassion for all beings, and extending that compassion into acts of kindness and understanding. In choices such as this, no one wins. To blithely dismiss the suffering of any being is contrary to Ahimsa.

Issues such as this require a deeper discussion. We need the sacramental acknowledgment of death that funerals and wakes provide; the grieving cycle with all its stages, the support of loved ones and society for that grief. Religious fundamentalists cannot claim the spiritual high ground when the decision is to give or take a life. Abortion is inherently a spiritual passage because it requires us to face the forces within us of life and death. Many argue against the legalization of abortion procedures, saying that humans have no right to choose who lives and who dies. But we have always been faced with such choices, and always will. The spark of the Supreme that resides in every being is fully capable of going deeper to find wisdom and healing, to discover the spiritual truth behind the events of our lives.

With the development of technology the decision to abort will be placed in the private domain, just as birth control already is, and abortion clinics will become a thing of the past. However, the ethics of choice will still be with us; abortion will remain a difficult and haunting choice, and until we face the spiritual dimension of that choice, the debate will remain what it is today — a dangerous, frightening, and destructive war of caricatures.

## THE RIGHT TO LIVE, THE RIGHT TO DIE

These times of advancing medical technology are forcing us to debate and, in many cases, to decide, questions of life and death. The opening of choice requires a level of consciousness that we feel unprepared for, and fear fuels debate into conflagration. Birth technology, including invitro fertilization, advanced methods of contraception, and abortion and genetic engineering, gives us difficult choices about life itself. We can save the lives of infants who, in another time, would have died at or before birth. It is conceivable that someday we may choose the sex and characteristics of our children; we may even forgo childbirth altogether in favor of an alternative birth technology.

These choices frighten us, and rightly so. Who has the power to give life, and to take it away? What sort of ethical consciousness will the lawmakers, healers, and scientists of the future have? Will money control matters of life and death? Science fiction and fantasy writers have given us glimpses of these advancements, and most often have painted a dismal and frightening future, with technology controlled by evil, materialistic megalomaniacs, corporations, governments, religions, and institutions. Few have given us visions of what it would be like if people of integrity — whose passion, purpose, and motive is love — guided the development and use of technology for the benefit of the earth and all beings. But we must try to envision it. The questions are important to ponder and discuss, even if we can find no answers now. Our children and their children will have to make ever more complex decisions and they need to grow up in an atmosphere of exploration if they are to be equipped to handle the future.

Undoubtedly, many of us have made difficult choices already, and were helped little by the legal system. Many of the shades of Ahimsa escape quantification and thus blur the boundary between law and conscience. What is legal and what is moral sometimes are not the same; often, legal standards follow moral ones, and good people are forced by circumstance to walk the line between.

How we die is becoming more and more a matter of human-chosen art and science, less an act of fate (I do not say an "act of God" because I believe God can act through human choices as well as through natural forces). Perhaps the most poignant in this regard are the questions of suffering. The AIDS crisis has confronted millions of people with death and dying before they ever thought they would have to face it. Advanced medical technology has enabled us to keep the body alive far longer than "nature" would. We now have to ask ourselves, "What is life?" Do we have a right to define it for ourselves? Do we have a right to define it for others? The questions are no longer theoretical but are clamoring for practical answers.

Derek Humphrey's book *Final Exit*, a manual for suicide for the terminally ill, sold nearly a million copies with no advertising, no author tour, and no reviews. Some people see the success of the book as a reason to despair about the state of our society. But it may be seen as a glimpse at our outrage at the medicalization of death, a wish for empowerment and choice, a fear of the loss of dignity and control at the end of our life's journey. In the 1970s millions of people began demanding dignity in childbirth, which led to the opening of birth centers, an increase in childbirth education and "natural childbirth," and fathers and families participating in the birth process; in general, a far wider array of choices and more in-depth education was offered than before. Now we turn our attention to that other profoundly important passage and question the intervention of technology and dehumanization of the death process. While 65 percent of Americans approve of voluntary assisted death for the terminally ill, legislation that would allow it has been defeated. We fear and distrust the medical and legal professions and their ability to provide assistance to us. These professions, which purport to exist for humanitarian service, are filled with technicians whose judgments are often skewed or overridden by money, power, and influence.

Humphrey favors legislation enabling physicians to assist those who wish to end their lives. He says, "Patients facing terminal illness, loss of control of life, and the end of quality in their lives should be permitted the compassionate assistance of a physician who can help to end a life with dignity." Opponents cite the "wedge principle," which maintains that by introducing an exception to the moral stricture against killing an innocent person, the door is open to abuse. They fear that institutional corruption would lead to the involuntary, compulsory killing of the poor, the aged, the mentally ill, and the handicapped.

If, as the yoga practitioners of the past have asserted, our integrity is like a muscle that grows stronger with careful exercise, it behooves us to grapple with these issues before they confront us. The process of grappling itself strengthens our integrity (our "Iccha Shakti") and thus we deal better with whatever we must.

It is not possible to live in the world and not commit some violence. But the intention to cause suffering can be explored. The value of practicing

Ahimsa is in becoming conscious of the pain we cause every day. We bring to consciousness those actions that hurt ourselves and others and choose (when it is possible for us to choose) to reduce those behaviors, to refrain from those acts, and to replace them with positive, life-affirming behaviors and attitudes. Eventually the practice of Ahimsa brings us to the state of mind in which we no longer have the impulse to do harm.

### AFFIRMATION OF AHIMSA

*I choose to behave with kindness toward myself, others, and the Earth. I choose not to, as far as it is possible, inflict pain or participate in the abuse of myself, other human beings, plants, animals, and the Earth.*

### (2) HONESTY — SATYA

Satya (pronounced "*saht*-yah") is speaking the truth with a spirit of kindness and living an honest life. Practicing Satya is about becoming whole and reclaiming the disowned parts of ourselves. Honesty is the only route toward wholeness, and wholeness is the real perfection.

Satya is not about becoming culturally perfect — becoming unreal, artificially rising above everything about us that makes us human. Perfectionism — an addiction that afflicts many of us and a web of lies that pervades our culture — is a kind of mask with attractive payoffs. It makes us feel entirely self-sufficient, so we fool ourselves into believing we do not need others (and thus do not need to be vulnerable to being hurt). It gives us a feeling of power, of being better than others ("an example") and allows us to judge, criticize, control, and correct others. Through a lens tainted with perfectionism, we view things as black and white, either/or, all or nothing. Thus we falsely simplify

Much pain comes from trying to be perfect. Perfection is impossible unless we think of it in a new way: Perfection is being who and where we are today.
— Melody Beattie

our lives and avoid the anxiety of difficult choices and gray areas. Perfectionism helps us avoid feeling dependent or needy, avoid trusting others, and avoid facing and accepting the unpleasant sides of ourselves.

Our culture promotes narcissism — the lie of perfectionism revisited. We are constantly assaulted by perfectionist images on television, in movies, and magazines. Women are particularly vulnerable to this attack. How many women are mentally and physically enslaved by the lure of the perfect body, the perfect face, the perfect hair, nails, and teeth? How many others must fight the demons of vanity and self-battering every day because they do not possess even the possibility of attaining our culture's idea of perfection?

I have never met a woman who has not endured this torture for at least a part of her life. And it is not "airheads" who think only about their desirability who suffer from this creativity-sapping obsession. Artistic, intelligent, powerful women who know better than to believe that physical perfection signifies their beauty suffer most from the barrage of lies from the media, from men, and from other women. There are many who profit greatly from this self-hatred and its resultant egocentrism. We spend millions of dollars every year trying to be perfect; entire industries are dependent upon our need to hide our imperfections and mask our humanness. What would happen if we were to become totally honest — genuinely, truly ourselves? How much energy would be freed up for creative activity, for real relationships, for spiritual fulfillment?

The real perfection is becoming a human being in the same way a tree is a tree. Satya is honesty that allows us to put down the burden of superficial perfectionism and join the human race.

Anger is sometimes a lie — it can often mask deeper feelings that are difficult to face. Dealing with anger in the spirit of Satya helps us go deeper. Rather than surrendering to the impulse to harm someone with words, we can spend some time discovering the pain that underlies the mask of anger. By observing the tightening of our defenses, the way we direct our feelings, and the moments that make up these experiences in the body and mind, we can bring a different kind of energy to them. As simple as it sounds, this is the stuff of intense spiritual practice.

Satya in our relationships with others means honesty and the right use of words with a spirit of benevolence. There is a difference between Satya and *rta*, which means objective, brutal truth. Satya means delivering bad news with an awareness of how that news will affect the person we are telling. It means protecting others who need our protection: for example, shielding an innocent person from an untrue accusation or giving support to the testimony of someone we know to be telling the truth, even when these actions are uncomfortable for us.

## SATYA IN PARENTING

Satya with our children means being as honest with them as is suitable for their age and who they are. It is not healthy to tell them everything about our lives, our inner processes, our fears, our relationships with others. But neither is it healthy to withhold ourselves from our children, or to withhold the entire adult world from them. Communicating with children involves a constant reevaluation of what is appropriate for them. They need a gradual midwifing into their adulthood so that they can start the process of being responsible, kind, and understanding people. It starts with being able to see their parents as human beings who suffer, who are sometimes confused, who

We look into mirrors but we only see the effects of our times on us – not our effect on others.

— Pearl Bailey

*155*

sometimes make mistakes.

Many of us grew up in households where an honest display of emotion was not allowed. Parents were not supposed to share their feelings with their children; parents were supposed to appear godlike, perfect, and strong. But this withholding of feeling doesn't work to bring people closer. Many people in my generation struggle to have an honest relationship with their parents now that they are older, and they resolve to be closer to their own kids. We have begun to realize that honesty is important to close relationships; it does not reduce our power, it enhances it.

When my son was a newborn baby, he was colicky. He hardly ever slept. I spent night after night awake with him. As I lost sleep I became more and more frustrated with his crying. It seemed that as I grew more frustrated, the crying became louder and longer. One night I found myself having fantasies of shaking him or striking him or throwing him out the window. Appalled at myself, I put him in his crib and went into the bathroom and cried. My pain at not being able to do anything for him and my frustration and exhaustion had reached its limit. As I sat and cried, I heard his cries from the other room. I began to think that perhaps contributing to my feelings of anger was my own withholding of my feelings from him, so that those feelings came to a point of extreme tension that could lead to battering. I suddenly understood how parents could become abusive.

I decided I couldn't be any more miserable than I already was, and neither could my baby. So why not share my feelings with him? I went to him and held him in my arms and began to walk back and forth as I had before. He cried, and I cried, too. I cried out loud; I cried as loud as he cried. We walked back and forth like that for around fifteen minutes, wailing and sobbing. Then he started to calm down and opened his eyes to look at me. I told him how frustrated I felt, how sorry I was that I couldn't do anything that would really help him, how much I loved him, and how terrible I felt that I had abusive thoughts. I told him all this looking into his eyes, and he seemed to be listening.

At that moment I stepped through a doorway into a relationship with my child that was to last a lifetime. From that point on, I listened to my child when he cried and I simply tried to be there for him in the way that I needed someone to be there for me when I cried. When I felt frustration and pain, I honestly let it show and shared it with him. This honesty has bonded us in a way that we both treasure. We've been able to share our lives, and while he respects me as his mother, he also knows that he has someone with whom he is safe — even in states of anger, fear, frustration, and pain. He knows his mom isn't perfect and doesn't expect him to be perfect. He knows it's okay to say "I'm sorry," and that struggle is a part of being human.

If children are to grow up being honest, and thus benefiting themselves and the world with the power of their integrity, they need honest models. They need to see us expressing our feelings honestly, owning up to our mistakes honestly, and telling the truth in all the little ways that compose the greater truth to which we aspire.

Dishonesty is not simply lying or withholding the truth. Dishonesty is expressed in numerous ways that undermine our integrity and personal power. Observing how each of these behaviors turns up in our expressions, we can bring awareness to them and begin to replace them with positive, healthy, honest ways of being.

Denial is acting as if we don't see the truth. It can be a healthy defense.

> What we say and what we do ultimately comes back to us, so let us own our responsibility, place it in our own hands and carry it with dignity and strength.
>
> —— Gloria Anzaldua

Women have always experienced the underside of patriarchy: the fist, the bottle, and sexual abuse. But with all our knowledge, women remain powerless against hypocrisy, rape, and abuse as long as we keep silent. The power of the Censor must be broken before we can become empowered.

— Starhawk,
*Truth or Dare*

It is the first stage in the grieving process, for example — a stage that helps us absorb the magnitude of a loss a little at a time. Denial is a shock absorber; it helps protect us from truths we cannot face. But in everyday life, denial leads to disharmony within ourselves and to family dysfunction.

We are taught denial in childhood when parents lie about what is happening. "Mommy's just tired" (Mommy's too drunk to stand up); "I fell down" (Daddy beat me up); "We're giving away the furniture so we can get a new set" (it's being repossessed because we're bankrupt). We thus learn that it's okay to lie about what is happening in order to fool ourselves and everyone else into believing that everything is all right. The payoff is that we don't have to face the magnitude of the pain the truth sometimes brings. The problem is that denial takes a tremendous amount of energy, like endlessly shoveling gravel into a bottomless pit. Underneath are the buried issues that control our lives.

We can break denial by allowing ourselves to become safe enough and strong enough to cope with the truth. Every day, in small ways, we can build strength and safety by taking care of ourselves and being honest with ourselves, by acknowledging what we cannot change and taking small steps toward changing the things we can.

If we grow up in an environment that prohibits or discourages an honest sharing of feelings and experiences, we never learn how to be honest appropriately. A no-talk rule may apply to one thing, such as sexual abuse or mental illness, but that one thing is connected to so many others that we must lie to ourselves and each other constantly just to uphold it. We can fool ourselves by thinking that as long as we don't talk about something, it doesn't exist.

## SATYA IN OUR SOCIAL AND POLITICAL CHOICES

When we follow Satya, we stand up for what we believe, regardless of the consequences. As we grow, change, and mature, our beliefs may change. What we are willing to risk for our beliefs may change as well, and every person has to evaluate this for him- or herself. "I speak the truth," Catherine Drinker Bowen said, "not so much as I would, but as much as I dare; and I dare a little more, as I grow older."

Honesty requires a deeply felt acceptance of ourselves and the gray areas of our lives. It is not possible to attain a life free of these gray areas, these hard places, the question marks wherein the truth can hide from us. Relativity always adds a little turmoil to the soup of life. The more deeply we are able to accept ourselves and others — to accept a little confusion — the more honest we can become. The more honest we become, the stronger our integrity becomes, and we find the strength to stand up for what is right when we know we must.

As we pare away the little lies, the bigger ones become less tolerable. It becomes more important to speak our truth in all our relationships, in our work and home life, and in our political choices. At the same time that life becomes less all-or-nothing, less black-and-white, it becomes easier to reach clarity within and act with honesty and forgiveness. In the spirit of this ethic, we think about our words and our actions and ask ourselves how honest we are being. We ask ourselves, "What am I willing to risk? How courageous can I be? Is this really right?"

A great part of Satya has to do with words, with putting our feelings into words. It is speaking from the heart. It is choosing words with care and with the intention of healing — with the intention of making the world a safe

> *Racism, classism and sexism will disappear when we accept differences and if we continue to resist loudly and clearly all racist, classist and sexist efforts on the part of other persons to enslave us.*
>
> — Martha Cotera

place for everyone.

Racial and sexual epithets diminish and demean and thus constitute a desperate effort to dominate and control. The words, the tone, the energy behind our language have tremendous power, and they require our attention if we wish to nurture our integrity. Sexism, racism, and cultural snobbery are built into our everyday language.

When we discover the ways our words disparage and humiliate others, often without our intending to, we may be tempted to throw up our hands. I once heard someone remark, "There's just no end to it! I'm so sick of people getting offended at every little thing. Why can't we all just be people?"

Rather than give up in frustration, we must try to find our way through to new words, new expressions, and new definitions that dignify and include. We must listen when others say they are hurt or offended by our words, whether we intended that hurt or not.

This effort to understand extends from our personal relationships into our communities, and can be a powerful force for change. The Rural Southern Voice for Peace (RSVP) was founded by Herb Walters in 1981 as a way to support activists in the South. Its Listening Project offers a way to use listening skills on a community level to help achieve lasting change and resolve conflicts nonviolently. Walters asserts that often activist strategies, such as debates, protests, vigils, legal action, and civil disobedience, polarize rather than unify when the component of compassionate listening is left out.

"With listening," Walters says, "you bypass the debate format and can overcome the barriers of defense and mistrust. When people feel safe, they challenge themselves. When you give people a chance to open up, they really examine their beliefs, and sometimes they reinvent them." The practice of

Satya includes a respectful attempt to understand the experience of others and use our own words to heal rather than harm.

## AFFIRMATION OF SATYA

*I am honest with myself today. I communicate my thoughts, feelings, and beliefs with kindness in all my relationships. I choose to speak and act with integrity.*

## (3) NOT STEALING OR WITHHOLDING — ASTEYA

Literally, (pronounced "ah-*stay*-ah") Asteya means "not stealing," which is simple enough. Asteya speaks directly to greed. When we choose to embrace this value in our daily lives, it starts with simply not taking what doesn't belong to us. Looking deeper, at what motivates us to steal, we come closer to the inner spirit of Asteya. Essentially, it is about withholding versus the ability to respond. We steal because we do not feel whole; when we do not feel whole we need to take from others and hold on to what we have.

Many people would consider Asteya a simple principle. Of course you don't steal — that's criminal. But how often are we confronted with a dilemma about withholding — money, material, information, love — and wonder what is right? When we are financially pinched and others are getting rich from cheating us, when we have deep concerns about survival, we may find ourselves justifying acts of withholding. We may not realize until later that we have diminished our innermost selves in the process. When we cheat on our income taxes, lie on an application for a loan, keep the wallet we found in the parking lot, or turn our face away from someone we love, our conscience throws up a warning. Each act of straightforward honesty builds our integrity. If we could see how these thoughts and behaviors change us —

how the light of our souls increases or diminishes — our choices would be clear. But we have all kinds of clever defenses against seeing the truth — defenses that help us maintain a convenient morality. Nobody wants to be a fool or a "goody two-shoes."

In our personal lives, Asteya is about choosing to be straightforward — to speak directly, to reveal ourselves, to ask for support or help when we need it. It involves respecting our own and other people's possessions, learning how to love others unconditionally and how to help others fulfill their needs. We meet our obligations, return the things we borrow, and clearly state our own conditions when we make agreements. This straightforwardness — called *rjuta* in yoga — is of fundamental importance in bringing the body, mind, and spirit into harmony.

## PARENTING WITH ASTEYA

Teaching our children responsibility begins with what *we* do. It is important that we make our struggles known to them, that we air our difficulties and dilemmas, that we allow our children to watch and participate with us in issues regarding honesty and straightforwardness. It is important that they understand that morality is not a commandment that you follow or you don't; rather, it is a constantly evolving aspect of our humanity, and a part of us that requires attention. Our understanding of what it means to choose not to steal will change as we grow; we will make mistakes and change our minds. Living with ethics is the process of being conscious about these choices, rather than simply reacting selfishly and impulsively.

Children can be taught, via stories, games, family discussions, and items in the news, the long-term consequences of cheating, stealing, or exploiting others. They can be taught the process by which we can come to decisions about what is right.

Opportunities appear every day to demonstrate to our children how to live responsibly. They can help with the recycling, save their outgrown clothes for a shelter, participate in road cleanup days, and help search for lost pets. They can be given age-appropriate household chores, with clear rules about how they are done, and clear, nonnegotiable consequences for not doing them (so chore-time doesn't turn into nagging and yelling sessions between kids and parents). It is not healthy to force kids to carry too much of the load, but children can be taught how to cook simple foods, how to do the laundry, and how to take care of animals and younger siblings. Praise and loving feedback instills in them a healthy self-regard and pride in their ability to be responsible. Feeling that they contribute in an important way to the well-being of others, kids learn more readily and acquire social skills of cooperation and peaceful coexistence. They are empowered to believe they can make a difference in this world.

## ASTEYA IN OUR SOCIAL AND POLITICAL CHOICES

Asteya has to do with boundaries: our personal boundaries, the boundaries in our relationships, and the boundaries of society. We all need to set limits, to choose what is healthy for us and what isn't, and to learn to respect others' choices. When we steal from others or when we withhold, we deny these limits. Boundary problems occur when they are either too rigid or nonexistent; healthy boundaries are permeable and lead to balance and a feeling of rightness.

Our society reflects our families' and our personal lives' confusion around

The enemy is our urgent need to stereotype and close off people, places and events into isolated categories. Hatred, distrust, irresponsibility, unloving, classism, sexism, and racism, in their myriad forms, cloud our vision so that individual and communal trust, responsibility, loving and knowing are impossible.

— Andrea Canaan

limits and boundaries. If a poor, African American man steals from a convenience store, he is sent to the penitentiary; a rich, white stockbroker embezzling millions pays a fine and is set free. Our immigration policy sets rigid boundaries for some and lets others in by the thousands; there is little sense to it.

Racism is a boundary violation, as is any expression of hatred or act of humiliation. An example of this is the controversy over the names of football teams. Native Americans have expressed dismay over names like "Redskins" and requested that these names be changed. Tim Giago of the *Lakota Times*, a weekly Native American newspaper in South Dakota, wrote:

> The sham rituals, such as the wearing of feathers, smoking of so-called peace pipes, beating of tomtoms, fake dances, horrendous attempts at singing Indian songs, the so-called war whoops and the painted faces, address more than the issues of racism. They are direct attacks upon the spirituality of the Indian people.... Stop insulting the spirituality and the traditional beliefs of the Indian people by making us mascots for athletic teams. Is that asking so much of America?

The management of these teams, however, asserts that the names are a tribute to qualities such as bravery and that the fans understand this — "lighten up," seems to be their position. Direct expressions of protest and requests for change from the very group the teams are named after are completely ignored — a clear violation of boundaries.

Many of the problems we face as a society have to do with boundary violations, the result of which is confusion and trauma. These include:

- Physical, emotional, and sexual violence in our families, our neighborhoods, and between races and nations.
- Disasters such as fires, tornados, earthquakes, hurricanes. (While we cannot control these, we can acknowledge and heal the boundary violations and their inherent trauma for those involved.)
- Pollution of the air, water, and earth.
- Using, torturing, and killing animals for food, clothing, and product testing.
- Abusing drugs, alcohol, food, and sex.
- An economy based on exploitation.
- Spying and covert "deals." (P. R. Sarkar once said that communism as a system leads to a society of spies; capitalism to a society of thieves.)
- Racism and sexism in advertising, sports, and entertainment.

Confusion means that which is fused together, a loss of clear distinction between one thing and another. Confusion reigns when boundaries are violated. To rationalize our own lack of boundaries by pointing to the corruption in our society only brings more confusion to the issue. If we are to free ourselves from confusion, we need to start with our own lives and set limits. We can choose not to be controlled by others. We can choose our values and choose to live by them. We can choose when to say "no" and when to say "yes," and we can choose to put off decisions until we feel clear about what we want. We can learn to live with the awkwardness and discomfort it sometimes causes when we set limits. The peace we feel inside when we know who we are and can feel a healthy pride in our values is worth it.

## AFFIRMATION OF ASTEYA

*I take responsibility for every aspect of my life. I can set limits and I respect the boundaries set by others. I choose to joyfully accept my obligations to myself, others, and the Earth.*

## (4) FOLLOW GOD, FOLLOW LOVE — BRAHMACARYA

The word Brahmacarya (pronounced "brah-ma-*char*-yah") means "to follow God." Its spirit is to accept that a higher power permeates every atom of the universe, and there is a universal rhythm — a "flow" — that goes on beyond our comprehension, in which everything is balanced and brought to order. The spirit of unity as an ethic of everyday life is to accept that God is love and that love is the force to which we can surrender our lives.

If we think of God as a mean-spirited, spiteful giant who extracts punishment for our sins, this surrender is certainly not a good idea! But a mean-spirited God is the God we make in our fear's image. When fear grows, it places limits on us and everything that comes into our world; we act with judgment and anger against ourselves and those we touch, and we place ourselves in hell. When love directs our lives — when our hearts are in charge — we act with mercy. Our world widens, becomes infused with beauty and tenderness, and we place ourselves in heaven.

We know in our hearts that God is love; we know that unconditional love is the result of something very great moving through our world. We recognize saints as those whose lives have become immersed in the energy of compassion and love for the whole universe as an expression of God, whose hearts and minds function as one, communicating that love through their words and actions. Unity means the unity of our hearts and minds. It is the process of allowing love to run our lives — the unity of the individual with the Supreme. From this place, everything we come in contact with is an expression of God that has its place and its reason. It gives us the ability to distinguish between love and fear, and to choose love more often than we choose fear.

There comes a time in our lives when something inside wakes up. Sometimes it is sudden, but more often it is a gradual stretching, slow-moving blooming that happens in tiny increments. It is the part of us that needs to find itself; our innermost being striving toward the perfect balance which is true humanness.

We may begin spiritual pursuits such as prayer, yoga, meditation, reading, and journal writing. Along with these, though, if our spiritual growth is to be meaningful in our everyday lives, we need to become conscious of our moment-to-moment process. By "process" I mean our physical, mental, and emotional patterns, feelings, and reactions. By observing ourselves with mindfulness, we can eventually begin to choose what we want to be and use our spiritual practices as tools to assist us.

We cannot take for granted that if we meditate in such a way, if we chant so many mantras, if we hang out with spiritual people, if we go to church regularly, we will magically become what we want to be. For without applying some consciousness to the moments of our everyday lives, without attention to our own unique set of internal beliefs and reactions, our spiritual practices only serve to keep us in one place. We may not go back, but we will not go forward.

This application of consciousness to the moment is Brahmacarya. There are many ways to practice this unity of mind and heart. One way is to begin removing the masks behind which we have hidden — perhaps since childhood. This can be painful, for it means we must feel our feelings, acknowledge much about ourselves that is not ideal, and speak and live the truth as it is for us. As scary as this can be, it is a practice that brings us into alignment with ourselves and thus closer to God. Maria Harris, in her book *Dance of the Spirit*, likens this to taking off makeup:

> It is the symbolic power of makeup that is really the issue. For cosmetics, which are probably the easiest masks to remove, are a symbol of all the masks we have learned to wear in public; masks that keep us not only from seeing ourselves, but also from being ourselves. Masks that keep us from our own aging or our own pain or our own beauty — or our own gaze.
>
> A much more constricting and damaging mask is the false expression we so often wear: of peaceful agreement when we are in raging disagreement; of pleasure when we are actually disgusted; of distaste when we are actually delighted; of humor when we are actually repelled; of understanding when we are actually baffled. We are so out of touch with our own feelings sometimes, that we have learned to produce what we know is the expected feeling. We are so intent on pleasing others ... that we learn to fake our reactions, and when we get really good at that, we learn to stop noticing our true ones.

How often have we lied with our masks? When does the mask appear, and how? What does it feel like? We can give ourselves permission to continue wearing our masks when we need them. At the same time, we can begin to allow ourselves to feel and identify what really happens when the mask appears. Meditation can help, for it develops the concentration necessary to observe ourselves with clear eyes and it keeps our minds engaged in the truth: that we are perfect expressions of the Supreme Being and there is no need to hide or lie.

Practicing the ethic of unity, we can begin, in small ways, to risk taking off our makeup: to be fully what we are in the moment, and to choose a loving way of looking at ourselves and at life. The result is serenity — a deep inner strength and peace, out of which the light of true joy can shine.

The most powerful way the practice of unity affects our lives is that it allows us to relax. In essence, it is faith and it is surrender. It is the most powerful and empowering step we can take — to let go, lighten up, stop trying to control everything, and start choosing to believe that a higher power is taking care of us and knows what it's doing.

As a young beginning meditator, I attended a yoga ashram where several people had recently received the instruction in this lesson of unity. One young man was particularly inspired about it, but hadn't yet realized its true meaning. He would stop before entering a building, close his eyes and look very holy for a minute. He would stop again before taking off or putting on his shoes, before eating, before getting up from the table, etc. It was amusing to watch him starting and stopping constantly. Nobody wanted to be around him because trying to interact with him was ridiculous. Before answering a question he'd close his eyes and look holy. Finally his meditation teacher saw him doing all this and took him aside, explaining to him that the practice of Brahmacarya was not an external show. He was instructed to try something more difficult: Continue your normal life, and allow yourself to feel love in every situation. When you eat, feel good about the food — enjoy its taste and texture, feel your gratitude and enjoyment, and know you are cared for.

*L*ove is a force in you that enables you to give other things. It is the motivating power. It enables you to give strength and power and freedom and peace to another person.

— Anne Morrow Lindbergh

When you talk to someone, relax, open up, really listen to what they have to say. When you put on your shoes, just put on your shoes! If you like your shoes, so much the better! These are the ways that unity of heart and mind are expressed. This is how we demonstrate that we recognize everyone and everything as an expression of God.

## PARENTING WITH BRAHMACARYA

For parents, a child's infancy is one of the easiest times to experience the feeling of unity. I remember the peaceful hours that went by, just watching my babies and being in love with them. As children grow up and begin asserting their separateness from us, we are required to bring this choice of unity to another level. We teach our children to trust their hearts by living from our own. And children require us to experience the pain of our separation more than anyone else. It can be very confusing, trying to be a healthy parent with our own childhood wounds. If we cannot find the child in us and begin to heal those wounds, we repeat what happened with our own parents. We project the child in us onto our own children, and react to their growth with fear.

My adolescent years were nonstop turmoil. Coming from a "broken," troubled home, I was a broken, troubled child with no self-esteem, no sense of personal boundaries, no trust in anything, and a lot of fear and shyness, which manifested as a mask of anger and rebellion. As my own children approached adolescence, fear started coming up for me again. I was lucky to have the sense and the support to work through my own buried issues in time to separate them from the reality of who my children really are.

When I was a young teenager, I was raped on a date. I never told anyone, because I felt deeply ashamed and blamed myself. No one would believe me or help me — in those days no one talked about it, and I knew it would be assumed that I was to blame. I became a "tough" kid, started taking drugs, stealing from department stores, and compulsively lying. There was no safe place for me. At home, I was battered by an alcoholic stepfather and spent nearly every night crying myself to sleep.

When my daughter wanted to start dating, my first reaction was "No way!" — not because I knew it was the wrong choice, but simply out of my fears. Remembering my own pain, I expected the worst for her. We sat down one day and talked about it. I began to see how different she is from who I was, how different her experience of life, the world, and relationships is from mine. I began to share some of my fears and experiences with her. "This is why I feel scared when I think about you going out with boys," I told her. I shared my story, not to scare her but to help her understand me. "I had some very painful times and I want to protect you, to help you see your choices and to support you. I need to work on seeing you for who you are, and trusting your good judgment, self-esteem, and healthy personal power. I hope you can work on understanding my fears and help me feel comfortable about your safety." When both of us agree to approach each other with love, we find a lot of room for us both to grow, to get our needs met, and to continue feeling unity as we separate to live our own lives.

## BRAHMACARYA IN OUR SOCIAL AND POLITICAL CHOICES

When we accept Brahmacarya as a value, it becomes the foundation for many of our social and political choices. If we believe there is an underlying unity to all things, and that unity is God or Spirit, to which we surrender our lives, it changes us. We begin to question the assumptions our society makes

*That Love is all there is,*
*Is all we know of Love;*
*It is enough, the freight*
*should be*
*Proportioned to the groove.*

— Emily Dickinson

about nearly everything. We begin to examine why we do or refrain from doing things. We begin to be concerned that, as far as possible, our choices reflect an awareness of the value we give peace and unity versus turmoil and separation.

I know many people who have turned away from lucrative careers that required turmoil, stress, and separation so they can choose to live peacefully, joyfully, and ethically. Struggle and pain will always be a part of life, but we have a choice about how that struggle will be lived — as a struggle against our deepest selves, or as a struggle to grow into wholeness.

The pain we feel when we reject love — and thus reject our own spiritual nature — is much greater and more destructive than the pain we feel in the process of surrendering our egos and our fear in a leap of faith. The one makes us hard and embittered; the other makes us soft and wise. We can refuse to believe the lie that only the mean, tough, hard, egoistic people survive and thrive. We can choose to believe that love is a greater power than any other can pretend to be.

Love is the basic survival requirement of every human being — even more so than food — and it is the energy that makes everything work. In the absence of love, things begin to go awry. Our fear of the great mystery of the unseen has driven us to accept a materialistic notion of the universe as a collection of particles of lifeless matter, and consciousness as little more than the result of chemical reactions in the brain. In separating from nature, we separated our minds from our hearts, and began to follow the dictates of the ego in its pursuit of limitless control. Thus emerged the industrial view of reality and its self-serving philosophy, which elevates greed to the status of a social virtue.

Each of us has work to do, a family to be a part of, a community in which we are involved, in one way or another. Each of us, choosing to act in ways that affirm the value of life, of love, of unity — no matter how insignificant or tentative these actions seem to us — has tremendous power. And the more people that make this choice, the more powerful the impact on our world. We don't need to risk our lives, careers, or families in this process; all we need to do is work on our intentions and follow our hearts. The rest will naturally unfold, bringing us and our world into harmony, into the experience of peace and unity.

## AFFIRMATION OF BRAHMACARYA

*Today I choose to believe in love. I release the fear that keeps me from feeling safe, supported, guided, and cared for. I dwell in my heart.*

## (5) SIMPLICITY — APARIGRAHA

The fifth "act of integrity" (yama) is Aparigraha (pronounced "ah-pa-ree-*gra*-ha"), simplicity.

While Brahmacarya is concerned with the subjective experience, Aparigraha is about our objective reality; the adjustments we must all make to the world around us. Yoga's definition of simplicity is not to allow greed to dominate our thoughts and actions. It addresses our acquisitiveness, and the importance of channeling that energy toward our emotional and spiritual well-being.

In our personal lives, simplicity is aligned with honesty. To be a "simple" person is to be clear, positive, and trustworthy, without angles and agendas, without deviousness, without guile. To find simplicity, we must first begin to look clearly at our lives and what complicates them. As we bring honesty into the forefront of our values, it becomes easier to see ourselves more clearly and to know when unnecessary stresses are bringing confusion and complication into our lives.

To live a centered life, one that is in line with our values, it may be necessary to find some time in which to allow all of the stimulation to stop, and allow our own thoughts to surface. When we are able to reach our own choices through meditation and contemplation, or by spending time in nature, it is much easier to find our priorities and stick to them.

How much of our lives are determined by what the media impresses upon us? How many of our choices are made because of a need to be politically correct, or to conform, or to gain others' approval instead of being made from our hearts' conviction? How much compromise have we chosen, and how much represents an erosion of our values by all of the stimulation around us? It may be difficult — but it is not impossible — to look at our lives and choices, to figure out what our priorities are and what constitutes, for us, the necessities of life.

To choose Aparigraha is to choose an outer life that is as much in harmony with our inner values as possible. To choose simplicity is to reduce the quantity while increasing the quality. It is to face the disease of greed as it has insidiously permeated our lives, and to make a daily commitment to its healing.

In our personal lives, we have many opportunities to choose simplicity — not because we "should," which implies not wanting to, but because we wish to live more compassionately. Simplicity is not self-denial, nor is it poverty; rather, it is choosing a different sort of richness. While poverty is involuntary, degrading, debilitating, and engenders despair, simplicity is chosen. It is enlivening, liberating, and it engenders empowerment. Choosing to live simply is to lighten, clean up, and streamline; someone once called it "living aerodynamically."

Some of the choices people have made in their personal commitment to simplicity include:

- Choosing products that are ethically produced.
- Participating in cooperatives — food, clothing, books, tools, repair, childcare.
- Developing skills that engender self-reliance: learning how to do home and car repairs, gardening, canning, cooking, sewing, and crafts.
- Participating in and developing extended family and support networks.
- Choosing products that are durable, functional, beautiful and non-polluting.
- Shifting diet toward vegetarian choices.
- Reducing clutter through sales and giveaways.
- Reducing overall personal consumption (clothes, jewelry, cosmetics).
- Choosing work that contributes to the well-being of self and society.
- Recycling.
- Investing in small-scale projects that contribute to personal and social well-being.

Twenty years ago, when I first began to work with the value of Aparigraha in my own life, I began looking around my environment with new vision. How much of what was in my life was necessary to the quality of my life and that of the Earth? One of the first things to become clear to me was the superfluousness of a meat-centered diet. If I could survive quite healthily as a

> The trouble with the rat race is that even if you win, you're still a rat.
>
> —— Lily Tomlin

vegetarian — and the choice rested with me — why did I find it necessary to participate in the torture and murder of animals? I had to look into my heart and ask myself if I really believed animals exist only for their utility value to human beings. I could not find any rationale for this position. When I looked into the eyes of an animal — whether it was the family pet, a cow, a deer, or a baby chick — and saw a sentient consciousness capable of responding, capable of feeling pleasure and pain, I could not convince myself that this being had no intrinsic, existential value, that it had no right to live its life.

So I adopted a vegetarian diet and gradually brought the ethic of simplicity into my life in other ways. It is a continuing process, with lots of loose ends. I am not the perfect vegetarian or the perfect animal rights consumer or the perfect ecofeminist or the model of simplicity. I've made mistakes and taken wrong turns. I have changed and my growth has gradually deepened my understanding of my own values. It has made the choices I make based on those values less automatic for me. Each day is full of tiny choices that, when consciously made, further my understanding and my ability to make the next choice.

It may at first seem that Aparigraha has little to do with our relationships. But the value of simplicity extends into every aspect of our lives. The clutter and accumulation of an unexamined life often includes energy spent on relationships that have little real value to us. To choose simplicity may require that we examine our relationships and what they mean to us. Do we spend lots of time on many superficial relationships to the exclusion of a few strong ones? How do we make priorities in our family relationships, our friends, our business associates? Have we chosen and nurtured a strong support network that will get us through troubled times?

At some point we each must realize that we cannot do it all. Each choice we make is not only a choice toward something; it is also a choice away from something. When we choose to accept every invitation to parties and social gatherings, we may be choosing not to spend quiet time with our families. When we choose to chauffeur our and others' children to every school event and extracurricular activity that comes up, we may be choosing not to have any creative time for ourselves.

Aparigraha is about examining our choices and embracing our choices *not to*. We choose what we want — that which will benefit us and our world in the long run — with a clear vision of what we don't want. We decide what we are willing to let go and what we wish to cultivate, and we pare our lives to the simple, elegant choices that make them rich with meaning.

## APARIGRAHA IN PARENTING

We can talk about all these issues with our children and help them to become aware of their own choices and how these choices ripple outward and have consequences in their lives.

Discussing purchases with our children (and making decisions about them together) can go a long way toward helping them feel secure and feel they are participants in, rather than victims of, the family budget. Arbitrarily restricting children's material possessions out of "principle" engenders resentment. But if a child can participate in some of the larger discussions about the money coming in and going out, he or she learns a tremendous amount about living in the world, about cooperation, and about getting one's own needs met while not neglecting the needs of others. Above all, children need to know that their worth is intrinsic; it does not depend upon keeping up with the material standards of their country, their school, or their neighborhood. This isn't learned simply by not allowing them to have the things other kids have. Rather, it is learned from their parents' attitudes and values as they are expressed in their words and actions in their own lives.

### APARIGRAHA IN OUR SOCIAL AND POLITICAL CHOICES

To choose simplicity is a radical move; it strikes at the very foundation of our economic structure. Our growth-oriented economy has brought us much-needed gains such as improvements in transportation, food production and distribution, and scientific research methods, and has raised our standard of living. However, it is time to reevaluate what is important to us. The growth economy is dependent upon the idea that more is always better. Thus, we have become enslaved to the rising and elusive standard of living as opposed to the quality of life.

The standard of living is measured in things and income; our quality of life is measured by people's well-being. In a growth economy one begins to push out the other. Our emphasis on economic growth undermines our sense of community and our feeling of belonging — in other words, our real sense of security. We are enslaved by the illusion that more things, more income will make us feel secure. And why not? We are deprived of the security of a community in which we have a valued place and on which we can depend in times of trouble.

A growth economy requires many components that undermine our real security and replace it with the false security of "getting ahead." It encourages individualism and competition over concern for others and cooperation. Our economy has reduced the sense of continuity and obligation in our families and engendered more dependence upon our individual resources and our ability to impress others. Thus, anyone who gets sick or falls behind is at risk.

Without community, we must win friends, seek relationships; we must influence people. The growth economy and its large corporations require mobility, so we must continuously reseek, remake, reimpress people over and over, never feeling secure in our relationships. And like our place in society, ideals of competition and individualism ensure that our relationships are always threatened in some way because they tend to depend more on what we do than who we are.

Everyone wants nice things and the freedom that wealth represents in our culture. But we also want to see the end of hunger and poverty. We want to ensure that everyone has a chance to live a life that is rich in significance, and in which the grinding pain of struggling for daily survival is removed. Research shows that a majority of Americans place a higher priority on human values and relationships than on material values and the standard of living. But until we begin making this priority we will never have the courage to stand up and ask the relevant questions of those whose greed runs our lives and contributes to destroying the lives of the twenty million people living in poverty in the United States.

We must take a look at what choices we have today, and start there. We can begin to live richly and simply. We can begin to change our drive for growth from the material level to the emotional and spiritual. We can lend our support to institutions, projects, and products that support our humanness, and to individuals who are engaged in life-affirming, cooperative behavior. We can build support networks that value people for who they are and that are committed to the security of the community. We can become educated and involved in our communities, particularly in decisions toward peace, unity, cooperation, and security.

### AFFIRMATION OF APARIGRAHA

*Today I choose to simplify my life. I now bring my values, words, and actions into harmony.*

## HEALTHY PRACTICES (NIYAMA)

The principles of Niyama help to build a lifestyle that supports the values of Yama. These are practical steps we can take to make our lives richer and more spirit-centered.

### (1) CLARITY — SHAOCA

Shaoca (pronounced "sha-*oh*-cha") is traditionally defined as "cleanliness." Through Shaoca, we get some sort of handle on the mess in our lives, both in a practical, physical sense and in the spiritual sense. It is possible to have a clean house and a messy, complicated mind. And it is possible to have a clear mind and a messy house — but not for long.

I define *Shaoca* as "clarity" rather than "cleanliness" because it encompasses the whole range of behaviors around the value of being clean, clear, simple, and direct. It's about cleaning the bathroom, but it's also about how our minds get cluttered with nonsense, how our world gets poisoned by the waste products of greed, and how all of these seemingly different things are connected.

Cleanliness is next to Godliness; it's true. However, Godliness may not always be next to cleanliness. While a saint may look at filth and see God, if you inspect her personal life you will find the utmost care for the cleanliness of her body and surroundings, even if those surroundings are in the worst slum in the world. You will find an orderly life, an orderly mind, and a sense of peace that comes through this basic value of herself.

I once spent some time at Mother Teresa's baby hospital in Calcutta, India, and the practice of Shaoca was apparent everywhere I looked. Each room was simple, aesthetically decorated, and clean. All the nuns and helpers were clean and had clear, direct faces. The hundreds of babies, lined up in group cribs that stretched from one end of the room to another, were clean and their linens were fresh. It was a safe and comfortable place to be. All this came out of Mother Teresa's love for God and her respect for everything and everyone as an expression of God.

In practicing Shaoca, first of all we pay attention to our bodies and our surroundings. Do they reflect a mind at peace? We needn't cultivate the controlling personality that shrinks in horror from a little dirt and spends hours ironing towels and scrubbing the tile with a toothbrush. Rather, we can check in with our bodies and take a look at our homes, cars, property, and workplaces now and then and ask ourselves if they truly reflect and support our state of mind. While we can learn to accept the mess of a "work in progress," taking steps to organize our workplaces and clean up our homes empowers us. It is yet another aspect of bringing consciousness to our choices and peace to our hearts.

Chinese philosopher Lao Tzu said, "He who values his body more than dominion over the empire can be given custody of the empire." Accepting clarity as a value, we keep our bodies and environment clean; we try to reduce the amount of garbage we produce and recycle what we can; we care for the beauty of our world and delight in creating beautiful, simple spaces in which to live our lives.

Just as dirt and clutter can destroy the serenity of our homes, selfishness, pride, jealousy, and rage can destroy the serenity of our minds. Embracing Shaoca means we commit ourselves to healing and thus "cleaning house."

Having clean, clear relationships takes work. It requires being honest all the time and having the courage to talk about what is in our hearts. When we live our lives trying to avoid pain, we take the crooked path. We don't realize that honesty is food for our spirits, and that our spirits begin to die of starvation when we begin to lie, to hide our true selves, to cover our feelings with a mask of invulnerability. Sometimes we need to move in the direction of pain in order to release it and find joy.

### SHAOCA IN PARENTING

With our children, Shaoca is more than bathing them every day and making them clean their rooms. If you watch children play in areas with and without fences, you will see that in a fenced playground they freely play in all the available space. They pop into the world of their imagination and explore. But without a fence, they clump together and fight, restricting the area they play in and avoiding the perimeters.

Children need the clarity of boundaries. The rules we set in our homes are like the fence; within these boundaries, they are secure and free to extend themselves. With no boundaries, they cannot explore; their spontaneity is limited and they either become fearful and withdrawn or reckless and aggressive. They will begin to act out in a subconscious effort to find the missing boundary line.

When boundaries do not exist, or when rules are arbitrary and enforced with rigidity, criticism, and shame, children grow up with boundary problems and find it difficult to know how to act appropriately.

Rules help children see where the "fence" that protects them starts and ends. There are both natural and logical consequences to all behavior. Logical consequences are those that are imposed when the natural consequences would be too dangerous or inappropriate. For example, the natural consequence of a toddler pulling the cat's tail would be getting scratched or bitten. But this is not a good risk for parents to allow. So a logical consequence needs to be clearly given by the parent. Logical consequences are best given in two or three stages. In this case, the parent could say, "No," physically remove the child's hand from the cat's tail, and show the child how to pet the cat gently, saying, "Kitties are for petting. Pet the kitty gently," smiling and rewarding gentle petting with strokes and kisses. If the behavior continued after a few of these efforts, the parent would move on to the next stage, saying, "No. Kitties are for petting, not for hurting," and remove the child from the cat. The third stage (depending on the age-appropriateness for the child) could be a time out sitting on a chair. Rules require both clear (but nonabusive), negative consequences for breaking the rules and positive consequences for succeeding.

Giving structure to our children's lives is one of the trials and gifts of parenthood. The more clean and clear we are able to be in all our communications, the more our homes will be safe places of serenity for our kids.

## SHAOCA IN OUR SOCIAL AND POLITICAL CHOICES

Embracing the ethic of Shaoca, we become aware of how we interact with our environment and what impact our personal choices have on it.

Politically, we can get involved in alternative solutions to local ecological problems and we can use the power of constituency to influence those who make the nation's policies. We can ask ourselves:

(1) How much garbage do I produce each day? What does it consist of? How can I reduce it? What measures has my community, my state, my country taken to address this issue? By using our food scraps for garden compost, recycling paper, plastic, glass, aluminum, and whatever else we can, we contribute a great deal to the future health and cleanliness of our communities.

(2) How much water do I use, and how much do I waste? Where does my water come from? How clean is it? What steps can I take to conserve water and ensure it will be clean and available in the future? Many futurists warn that a global water crisis is inevitable if we do not begin to pay attention to how we use and misuse this precious gift of life.

(3) How much of what I own serves a valuable purpose in my life? How much is unnecessary and not of use to me? A good way to clean up our homes is to recycle the clothing, tools, kitchen items, toys, and other "stuff" we no longer use by donating them to charities that can repair and give or resell them to others.

(4) How clean is the air I breathe? What steps can I take to reduce air pollution, both inside and outside my home?

(5) Are there environmental hazards in my region? How can I effect change and help protect my area from these hazards?

(6) Is there beauty and simplicity in my life? How do I feel in the atmosphere and physical setting of my home, my vehicle, my property, my workplace? Does it enhance my mental peace? What steps can I take to change my environment so that it does so? Can I introduce artwork or other objects to beautify it? Would plants or animals like to share my space and add to its wholeness and balance? (And can I commit to serving them?) Can I change the color or lighting or introduce soothing fragrances? Can I reduce clutter and thus increase clarity? Is there a special place I can go to meditate and nourish my spirit?

## AFFIRMATION OF SHAOCA

*Today I choose to be clean and clear in thought, word, and action. I behave with clarity in all my relationships. I contribute to the beauty of my world.*

## (2) ACCEPTANCE — SANTOSA

*Tosa* means a state of mental ease. Santosa (pronounced sun-*toh*-sha) is the contentment that comes from accepting ourselves and others just the way we are. It is not a passive denial of our power; it is not a surrender to fear. Rather, Santosa is the practice of choosing love over fear in our everyday lives. Fear and all its accompanying reactions goads us into frantic activity or drags us into frozen depression. When we realize we have a choice, and when we make that choice toward love, our lives come into balance and we begin to feel contented.

The joy that is the result of practicing acceptance can only be ours when we begin with ourselves. If we do not accept ourselves at this moment, we cannot access love in our relationships or for the betterment of our world.

Acceptance is the magic that makes change possible.

— Melody Beattie

Self-acceptance is not an easy practice in a dysfunctional society. The mirrors we face every day — on television, in magazines, at work, in the marketplace — stare back at us with disapproval. We can never be thin enough, rich enough, smart enough, successful enough, or even happy enough! When we react to this pressure from our own unhealed pain, we feel driven, desperate, and unhappy. Happiness is just out of reach; perfection is just around the corner. Serenity is out of the question.

Practicing Santosa in our relationships requires that we accept the things we cannot change, we change the things we can, and we learn the difference between the two. A relationship is always changing because we are always changing. Our relationships have the power to teach us the most important lessons we came here to learn, and so the more intimate and committed a relationship is, the more it teaches us. Even passing acquaintances can help us practice acceptance and thus allow the light of peace to shine from our eyes. An encounter with a sales clerk or a police officer or a mail carrier mirrors our consciousness and gives us another chance to bring love and healing to the world.

Acceptance is a powerful attitude. We can accept a situation and yet work to change it. We can accept others and still have choices about our relationship to them. Sometimes we mix up acceptance with denial. A woman who "accepts" the abusive behavior of a violent spouse has not accepted him; rather, she is denying the truth. When she truly accepts the fact of the abuse, she can choose to get out and get help.

Practicing Santosa in our intimate relationships helps us learn to influence rather than control. We learn not to load others' behavior with so much "charge"; we learn to negotiate and compromise to get our needs met and to help our partners meet their needs. We learn to ask ourselves, "How important is this?" We learn to roll with life, to accept others' foibles, failings, idiosyncracies, and fears. Life is no longer a crisis because we choose contentment.

> Courage is the price that life exacts for granting peace.
>
> — Amelia Earhart

## SANTOSA IN PARENTING

Practicing Santosa with our children helps them grow up feeling secure and loved, with lots of healthy personal power and self-esteem. Young children need to be cared for, to be touched and told they matter. They need to be noticed and accepted exactly as they are.

Sometimes parents, under the influence of our own woundedness, think that our job is to straighten our kids out. So every communication, every instance of eye contact, is charged with shame, humiliation, disapproval, correction, and criticism. This is all well-intentioned; most parents want to do the right thing and are fearful of doing wrong, so that our children don't "turn out right." What we don't realize is that belittling, pushing, criticizing, or neglecting behavior is deeply harmful to our children and has the effect of making them into exactly what we fear.

Santosa is unconditional love. It says, "I love you because you are here. I am glad you are my child. You deserve love; no strings attached." Both abuse and neglect interfere with a child's development and perpetuate the chain of pain. Wounded children are wounded adults, who hurt themselves and others and contribute to the making of a cold and violent society.

## SANTOSA IN OUR SOCIAL AND POLITICAL CHOICES

Santosa enables us to find a perspective when we are dealing with social and political injustice. Some social activists reject spirituality because they fear that it might engender a passive acceptance of exploitation; indeed, religious dogma has given rise to such passivity and to its opposite as well — rigidity that leads to war. But true spirituality and a practice of Santosa are not rigid or passive.

Practicing Santosa, we allow ourselves to face reality and accept it. We fight injustice not out of fear, anger, and revenge, but with a love that gives us courage. When Christ admonished his followers to "turn the other cheek," I believe he meant that we must work to stay centered when we are threatened with aggression, oppression, and exploitation. When we do not allow ourselves to get sucked into the fear that such a situation generates, we can act with courage and resolve to protect ourselves, our loved ones, and the earth from those whose pain has caused them to act out the ego's fearful dreams. Without the awareness of Santosa, we are easily pulled into the same negative energy we are fighting against. Santosa is the practice of making ourselves quiet so as not to be at the mercy of our anger, our outrage, our feelings of injustice.

When we live every day with the act of faith in a higher power, when we choose not to succumb to fear, every circumstance in which we find ourselves enriches and strengthens us. When bad things happen, it is those whose love is strong and clear, who are capable of accepting truth and acting with faith, on whom others rely.

## AFFIRMATION OF SANTOSA

*Today I choose to be contented. I accept myself and I accept others as they are. I accept the world as it is, and choose to contribute to its healing.*

## (3) GIVING OF OURSELVES — TAPAH

Tapah (pronounced "*tah*-pa") has undergone several incarnations in its definition. In Patanjali's time, Tapah implied the mortification of the body to reach higher states of consciousness. Yoga practitioners would sit in freezing water or in painful postures or would fast in an effort to rid themselves of the attachments of the physical body; many Christian monks and nuns did likewise. This is where the image of a yogi on a bed of nails came from. But later interpretations — including Buddha's great contribution to the world — rejected these practices because they merely replace the attachment to pleasure with the attachment to pain, creating an unnatural aversion to everything that makes us human.

With later interpretations of Patanjali's work, Tapah came to be seen in a more positive light, meaning "self-discipline" or "self-restraint" — the attainment of a kind of self-sufficiency that allows yoga practitioners to release their attachments and thus rid themselves of greed. But too much self-sufficiency is a kind of greed in itself. We are all part of a universe that requires our participation, our interdependence with other beings.

Practicing Tapah keeps us aware of our connection with others. In American society the word "sacrifice" implies a kind of sickness. We detest self-righteousness and the martyrdom of people who are enslaved to taking care of everyone but themselves. However, in healing ourselves of the compulsive other-centeredness of codependency, we sometimes throw out the baby with the bath water, becoming more and more self-centered as we replace an obsession with pleasing others with obsessively taking care of ourselves.

Middle-class life offers very little opportunity for children to learn the joy and the pain of serving their less fortunate brothers and sisters. In many third world cultures the children participate in the struggles of daily life. Their observation of their parents' sacrifices for others imbues in them a sense of human obligation to help, and with it, a trust in the natural order of things.

American culture has little or no opportunity or support for this type of participation and learning. Suffering, deprivation, and pain are sanitized and removed from our experience so that we view those who suffer with an aversion and a pity that keeps us distant. With no daily relationship to suffering, the fear of it grows large and we work frenetically to keep "the wolf from the door." Because we have created a society in which we can live our entire lives not knowing our neighbors we have won freedom from social bonds — we have gained the privacy of individuality. But the price we have paid is dear.

Defending ourselves against the suffering of others, we have invited another kind of suffering — that of loneliness, isolation, and despair. And we have not gained security or safety in our isolation; suffering will come to us no matter how many walls we build around ourselves. If the pain of those who suffer from injustice doesn't come to burn down our homes or businesses, most of us will still have to face old age and illness without the security of a community that respects and cares for us. This is the nature of fear-based living; the very walls our egos build for protection become the prisons in which our spirits languish.

Practicing Tapah — giving of ourselves to serve those in need — is one of the most powerful spiritual practices available to us. It awakens our hearts to our connection with others; it mirrors our unhealed places and gives us the opportunity to grow; and it gives us the chance to feel the support, the love — the energy — of our higher power in our lives.

Tapah is the act, however small, of quietly giving beyond what normally and naturally comes to us. It is not the routine writing of checks to foundations for the poor; nor is it the grandiose gesture that gets our name in the newspapers. It is neither other-centered nor self-centered. The secret of real Tapah is that it is done without any fanfare, it is done through sacrifice, and it is done simply for the sake of doing it.

Practicing Tapah does not require us to go to Calcutta to work with Mother Teresa's Missionaries of Charity. We can find plenty of opportunities to practice right in our own backyards. We don't practice Tapah because we feel it is an important thing to do or that we are making a big difference. It is done simply because it is a part of being on this Earth. Some of the ways Americans have found to practice Tapah include:

- Making a commitment to help someone we know who is ill or injured.
- Participating in "meals-on-wheels" projects in which we have a chance to connect person-to-person with the people we are serving.
- Volunteering at a shelter for the homeless, for battered women, for abused and abandoned children, for people with AIDS, at a hospice for the dying.
- Volunteering to help with a local food distribution center, or starting one ourselves.
- Being a foster parent or a "big brother" or "big sister."
- Teaching others to read through a literacy program.
- Volunteering on a hot-line service for suicide prevention or child abuse.
- Getting paramedical skills and volunteering in an ambulance, fire, or disaster service.

Tapah can include donating food, clothing, or money to causes that help those in need, but real Tapah requires us to face those we serve and to interact with them. It is sometimes very difficult to find time to serve others in this way; with family and career responsibilities, there are only so many hours in a day. For some, taking time off to do service works better; we may volunteer for a year in the Peace Corps or take vacation time to work in a service project full time. When we are open to them, opportunities to grow through sacrifice come to us; we don't need to look very far.

## TAPAH IN PARENTING

Children are the best teachers of Tapah we can possibly have. In order to be good parents we must be willing to sacrifice for our kids; to stretch ourselves beyond our fear and limitations. Walking the baby all night long, changing diapers, developing routines in which our children can feel safe and protected, planning for their education, providing medical care, emotional support, boundaries and freedom — all require us to give of ourselves, to reorganize our lives and our priorities. Parenting goes wrong when the spirit of Tapah is lost and fear takes over.

One of the important reasons teenage pregnancy is often a tragedy is that two very powerful forces of growth are required at the same time, and this double-bind is nearly impossible to negotiate. The teenage years are a time of individuation, when the ego goes into full swing because of the fear generated by separation from parents and home. It is thus a time when we are selfish and self-centered; we have a difficult time understanding others and giving of ourselves for their welfare. When individuation has been achieved and our fears are assuaged, we're ready to put our spirits back in the driver's seat and to grow through sacrifice.

The core requirement of good parenting is the ability to place a child's needs ahead of our wants, and to feel safe and centered ourselves so that we can provide safety and balance to our children. How can a teenager possibly achieve both of these phases of growth at the same time? It's no wonder that children of teenaged parents are often abused and neglected.

Altruism is defined as an unselfish regard for or devotion to the welfare of others and behavior that may not be beneficial to oneself (or may be harmful or risky) but is done for the benefit of others. Thus, it is a key character trait for the development of Tapah, which is similar in definition but includes a spiritual component — that of embracing humanity as an expression of one's deepest Self, or God.

Social scientists have studied altruistic people in order to develop educational environments to foster and support volunteers in various social service arenas. In one study, two groups of former volunteers in the civil rights movement were studied. One group consisted of those who were partially committed — who participated in one or two freedom rides or demonstrations. The other group consisted of fully committed activists who had worked continuously for over a year in the movement. The most significant differences between these two groups centered around their experiences in childhood, and specifically, their relationship with parents.

The partially committed group members were more likely to have negative or ambivalent relationships with their parents, who preached altruism but did not practice it. These people reported parental hypocrisy and described current relationships with their parents as cool and distant.

The fully committed, on the other hand, tended to have involved, nurturing parents who modeled altruism in their own lives. They admired their

A Woman's Guide to Tantra Yoga

parents and described their current relationship with them as close and warm. In addition, these people were what researchers termed "autonomous altruists;" that is, their desire to serve was internally directed, while that of the partially committed tended to be motivated by external rewards (the approval of peers, etc.).

Subsequent research has borne out these findings, and gives us some guidelines for developing a consciousness of empathy and service in our children. While we must remember that our children have their own soul-plan that we do not determine for them, providing an atmosphere that encourages the growth of an unselfish character can support them in developing that plan. Elements of this environment include:

(1) A responsive attitude from parent to child that includes lots of demonstrations of love and affection.

(2) An empathic response from parents that communicates understanding and respect: "I want to know how you feel; I understand how you feel; I respect how you feel."

(3) A modeling of altruistic behavior by parents toward others that is not at the expense of attention to the needs of the children. When children hear their parents discussing an injustice then see them trying to do something about it, they will emulate that behavior in their own adulthood.

These three guidelines seem simple, but they can be very difficult to carry out if we have not healed ourselves. Our hearts are like chalices, meant to be filled with unconditional love. When filled to overflowing, we naturally turn outward toward others, and we are not depleted or made ill by selflessness. But if the chalice is not filled, we feel a vacuum, an emptiness. We seek to fill this void and, quite naturally, every act of love is a selfish one.

To fill our children's hearts so that they may touch many others with true, unselfish compassion, we must heal our own emptiness at the same time. We cannot wait, because in waiting we doom our children to repeat the same pattern. In the yoga tradition, this fulfillment is attainable by actively seeking unity with and guidance from our deepest spiritual core. We can enlist our will and our spirit to choose fulfillment. We can choose to pass that fulfillment on to our children through conscious commitment to their welfare and by modeling the behavior we wish to see in them. Perhaps in this way, several generations down the line, empathy, love for humanity, and selfless service will be "traditional" in our families and a part of what we consider to be good mental health.

## TAPAH IN OUR SOCIAL AND POLITICAL CHOICES

Tapah is often called "selflessness," but this term has a negative connotation in Western society. It is not so much about being selfless as it is about practicing the release of our fears; it is *egolessness*. It is not about losing ourselves in others, or neglecting our own needs, our mental peace, or our health to be there for other people. Occasionally, this "emergency" mode of service is required; an accident or a disaster may require temporary service from us in which we completely put aside our normal lives and our everyday needs. However, if we find ourselves in a lifestyle of emergency and crisis, something is wrong. We can practice sacrifice as a part of our everyday lives, just as we practice clarity or acceptance.

Politically, we have come to value cleverness more than sincerity. The media portrays a sincere politician as stupid and encourages admiration of those who are smooth and can give seamless performances. We have come to take for granted that a politician must be selfish, greedy, and business-like. Politics is currently a business career, not one of service. We expect a politician to do things only because they serve his or her own career.

At some point we will begin to use human values as a measuring stick: How has this candidate demonstrated honesty in his or her professional and personal life? How congruent are his or her words and actions? And finally: Does this candidate have experience in service? Has he or she sacrificed for others less fortunate? Does he or she demonstrate an ethic of service when the cameras are not rolling?

## AFFIRMATION OF TAPAH

*Today I open my heart to myself and others. I am willing to extend myself in service to someone in need. I trust my higher power to guide me.*

## (4) UNDERSTANDING — SVADHYAYA

In ancient India, Svadhyaya (pronounced "swad-*yah*-yah") was the study of spiritual scriptures. It implies the use of the mind to understand how the universe works. It is much more than reading books or listening to sermons; it is true understanding, which requires an effort to grasp the underlying significance of spiritual ideas, and using our rational judgment in concert with our feelings and intuition.

Understanding, as a spiritual practice, is a commitment to the truth. We learn to listen and to read with our hearts, and to use our minds to filter out the garbage and find the gems. Every religion, every spiritual teaching has gems of true knowledge. But these are often cloaked in the dogma that armors the egos of so-called religious people driven by fear. Daily spiritual practice — and particularly deep meditation — sharpens our intuitive faculties and helps us see through this armor.

We can follow any spiritual path we choose; it is our understanding that will bring us enlightenment and peace, not the rote practice of one discipline or another. We take ourselves into heaven or hell by choosing whether our hearts or our egos will run our lives. The mind is like the very best of tools: in the hands of an artist it can create beauty; in the hands of a homicidal maniac, it can destroy life. When the mind is used by the heart, with compassion, we grow in knowledge and understanding. When the mind is used by the ego, with fear and hatred, we grow hard and our world contracts.

I have always thought of Svadhyaya as the practice of fine-tuning what I call my "nonsense sensor." It's that radar-of-the-heart that tells me something's wrong. It tends to go off when I hear or read something that makes no sense; something that condemns, judges, or maligns; something that sounds like fear masquerading as spiritual or religious teaching. Meditation can sharpen this faculty if it is done wholeheartedly, with consciousness. Reading spiritual books can give us practice in understanding our own spirituality and broadening our perspective. Svadhyaya is the practice of looking deeper — within ourselves and the world around us.

## SVADHYAYA IN PARENTING

I worked with parents and infants for twenty years, teaching massage techniques as a way to strengthen relationships. Through this daily contact with parents and infants I discovered that the one and only problem infants have is not being heard. Massage became a vehicle through which I could help parents learn how to listen to their babies. When an infant is finally listened to wholeheartedly, everything changes. Colic clears up, the baby relaxes and begins to really shine with his or her inherent joy. Most people don't realize that babies have as much to talk about as we do, and that they need to ventilate emotions and have their feelings received with love and acceptance. So do children. And so do adults. But often we respond by hardening our hearts, armoring for war. Someone else's pain can trigger fear and a reminder of the anguish and rage we may have felt as children, crying alone in a crib with no response, unable to express negative feelings and have them received. It can also engender guilt (Am I a bad person if I caused this pain?) that often leads to anger and revenge as our egos try to defend against a perceived attack.

Learning how to listen with our hearts is one of the most valuable contributions we can make to our relationships — including our relationship with ourselves. A listening heart provides an atmosphere in which exploration of all the layers can take place.

## SVADHYAYA IN OUR SOCIAL AND POLITICAL CHOICES

In our social lives, Svadhyaya is that which brings us a deeper knowledge and understanding of social and political forces. The media reduces all our news to the lowest common denominator — to either-or and all-or-nothing choices — and so we find ourselves taking simplistic stands on issues about which we have little information. Svadhyaya is the refusal of the simplistic; it is the effort to get the information and make rational choices. It is the process of listening to what social leaders and politicians are saying between the lines, and applying human moral standards to our beliefs. Racism, sexism, ageism, injustice of any kind is a product of fear. When we react with fear rather than responding with love and understanding, war breaks out.

We all fear the hard realities of where our society is headed, because in our hearts we know that what goes out from us comes back to us. There are no longer any simple answers to our social problems; enormous changes will have to happen before we can begin to grow healthy again. Our economic system is destroying our environment, and saving our environment will require a total restructuring of our way of life. Providing a healthy environment for every human being, plant, and animal must eventually become our one and only mission, for which we are willing to change the way we live right now. Practicing Svadhyaya — reading, listening, trying to understand the truth — can help us individually change in ways that support the healthy change of our communities and our world.

## AFFIRMATION OF SVADHYAYA

*Today I seek a deeper understanding of life. I am willing to see things differently. I read and listen with an open mind and heart in order to form compassionate, responsible opinions.*

## (5) SPIRITUALITY — ISHVARA PRANIDHANA

Ishvara Pranidhana (pronounced "eesh-*war*-ah pra-nee-*da*-na") is a mouthful; let's use the term *spirituality*. The literal meaning of the Sanskrit is "to take shelter in the Supreme." This, to me, connotes a joyful surrender — a decision to make spirituality the point and purpose of our lives. Spirituality

Any God I ever felt in church I brought in with me.

—— Alice Walker,
*The Color Purple*

is both a value in itself and a result of choosing kindness, simplicity, honesty, acceptance, responsibility, unity, clarity, sacrifice, and understanding in our everyday lives.

Spirituality can be expressed in many ways. In the yoga system, spirituality is both a practice and a sense, or feeling, about who we are that comes out of that practice. Time-tested techniques include yoga postures, which refine the body; healthy food, which calms and strengthens both body and mind; meditation, which refines the mind and nurtures the heart; and ethical behavior, which brings our hearts and minds together in relation to others and our world.

When spirituality is the core of our lives, it is as if a loving parent is watching over a growing child. It is said that the mind (and its outward expression, the ego) is a terrible master, but a wonderful servant. The only way to appropriately use the mind is to put our hearts in control of our physical, mental, emotional, and spiritual well-being. In this context I equate the heart with what we may call soul or spirit: the aspect of our being that is in harmony with unconditional love.

Setting aside time each day to pray or meditate in solitude helps us bring awareness to the rest of the day. Quieting the mind and directing its flow toward oneness with the inner Self allows us to reexperience the peace and joy that is the heart of all existence. Accessing this inner connection helps us to behave in ways that reflect our values, and thus our impact on the world around us is positive and profound.

One of the most useful projects I have undertaken is to write a "mission statement" for my life. I did this several years ago, and every year on New Year's Day I review my statement and make any changes I need to make to bring it into alignment with what I understand to be my chief purposes. I also review the past year, and evaluate what I have done and how I have expressed my stated mission in my everyday life. If there is an area that is being neglected, I try to understand why and figure out how I might address that aspect in the coming year.

My mission statement consists of my guiding principles: statements, in my own words, about how I wish to be in every area of my life. Throughout the year, as I plan all my activities and goals, I review this statement and ask myself, "Does this project, plan, or goal resonate with my mission in life?"

You may already have an overall statement of purpose about being a good person, or realizing God, or serving humanity, or whatever. Breaking that general purpose down into specific behaviors can be very helpful. You will find yourself doing more thinking, less reacting. We are pressured, cajoled, manipulated, and maneuvered into doing countless things that don't necessarily move us any closer to our goals, and that may, in fact, pull us away from our fundamental principles. Stating these principles can be the first step toward gaining the inner strength and courage to be what we really, truly want to be, deep-down in our souls.

When you have finished your statement of purpose, you may want to frame it and put it where you can read it for inspiration each day. Whenever you plan your year, your month, your week, or your day, review your statement first, to be sure all your activities contribute to your personal mission in life. When you have stated concretely what is most important to you, it is a lot easier to say "no" to things that are extraneous to it.

It is important, when doing this exercise, to be completely honest with yourself; forget about what you are "supposed to" feel, think, and do. This mission statement will be of no use to you if you do not write it in your own words, from your own heart, reflecting who you are and what you want. If "selfless service to humanity" is a life purpose for you, how can you express that in words that make sense to you right now? What are you doing right now that reflects this purpose? In what specific ways can you express this purpose in your behavior toward others who are closest to you? If you are not expressing this purpose, why not? In some cases, you may discover that you have been given a purpose by someone else and you have never really made it your own. This is a time to reevaluate those preprogrammed ideas and discard what doesn't resonate deeply with you right now.

It is easy to see what is wrong; it takes practice to notice what is right. We must learn to identify and accept reality — but because we have been taught to see the world with fear, we often become habituated to equating reality with negativity. When we begin to see the world and our lives through the eyes of love we understand that joy is the fundamental reality of all existence, and that love can empower us even in the most painful times. Fear and hatred can be released.

It is natural for us to feel pain sometimes, to experience negative emotions, to know the dark side of ourselves and our world. Denying this dark side keeps us from learning and growing. When we cannot feel intensely negative, we cannot feel intensely positive either; denial leads to frozen feelings and an inability to empathize with others. It is a kind of "positive negativity." But we can take the next step — into a positive, joyful way of seeing — and bring ourselves back into harmony. Negativity takes us out of harmony and gives power to our problems.

Choosing positive energy, we empower ourselves to find healthy solutions.

Because we believe in love, we can face hatred. When we are no longer controlled by fear, we enter a new reality, where joy is an everyday feeling. We begin to notice all the beauty around us. Expressing and receiving love and support, we become accustomed to feeling safe and cared for. We move swiftly through sad feelings and problems as we become successful at negotiating life's terrain. Like expert sailors, we learn how to handle the storms and dangers — and we learn to love the sea. Pleasure, fun, enjoyment, laughter, intimacy, and spiritual joy — all become the reality of life for us.

## SELF-ANALYSIS

Honesty makes room in our hearts for ourselves and each other. Once a week, we can take time to make a personal inventory of our lives and look bravely at our mistakes and behavior. An art teacher once said to me, "There is no such thing as a failure. Rather, we are successful at learning what we don't want to repeat."

Admitting we have behaved in a way we regret, or that we have made a mistake or unintentionally hurt someone helps us move into healing and joy. This can be threatening to our egos, which are fearful of being vulnerable. If we were shamed as children, feelings of shame may arise when we make mistakes. Instead of the healthy remorse out of which comes healing and change, we struggle with self-hatred. Shame breeds anger as the ego strives to protect us from the pain of self-annihilation. We put ourselves and others out of our hearts and the damage remains. Looking at our mistakes with kindness and courage, we become truly human. How often have we wished that someone who hurt or disappointed us could just acknowledge our pain and sincerely say, "I'm sorry"?

Regular self-analysis teaches us appropriate humility and makes room in our lives for growth. We can use Yama and Niyama or our Personal Mission Statement as a guide for our inventory, discovering where we have unconsciously chosen fearful reactions when we could have chosen love. We can look for the ways in which our feelings, thoughts, and behavior have reflected old patterns. We can also discover ways in which we have been successful at seeing the world with love. We can look for the ways in which our feelings, thoughts, and behavior have reflected trust, faith, courage, self-esteem, honesty, unity, and understanding. Self-analysis is not to punish ourselves for wrong-doing; rather, it is a way to lovingly parent ourselves into wholeness.

## COUNT THE BLESSINGS

Consciously noticing all the good things empowers our lives with healthy positive energy. Each night before we go to sleep, we can take an inventory of all the good things that happened during the day.

We can ask ourselves what is right, what is good, about our behavior and feelings, other people, our work, our relationships, our world. Wouldn't it be great if the evening news included at least equal time for good news? Since it doesn't, we can provide ourselves with good news each evening, and go to sleep feeling blessed. Melody Beattie, author of *The Language of Letting Go*, writes about this beautifully:

> Gratitude unlocks the fullness of life. It turns what we have into enough, and more. It turns denial into acceptance, chaos to order, confusion to clarity. It can turn a meal into a feast, a house into a home, a stranger into a friend. It turns problems into gifts, failures into successes, the unexpected into perfect timing, and mistakes into

important events. It can turn an existence into a real life, and disconnected situations into important and beneficial lessons. Gratitude makes sense of our past, brings peace for today, and creates a vision for tomorrow.

## AFFIRMATION FOR IISHVARA PRANIDHANA

*May all beings dwell in the heart. May all beings be free from suffering. May all beings see the bright side of everything. May all beings be healed. May all beings be at peace. May God's will be done.*

---

Recommended Reading:
*A Guide to Human Conduct* by P. R. Sarkar
*Everyday Ethics* by Joshua Halberstam
*The Woman's Book of Confidence* by Sue Patton Thoele

*S*pirituality is not a utopian ideal but a practical philosophy which can be practiced and realized in everyday life. Spirituality stands for evolution and elevation, not for superstition or pessimism. All divisive tendencies and group or clan philosophies that create shackles of narrow-mindedness are not connected with spirituality and should be discouraged. Only that which leads to broadness of vision should be accepted.

— P. R. Sarkar

# Chapter Seven
# Changes

*In the house with the tortoise chair*
*she will give birth to the pearl*
*to the beautiful feather.*

— Aztec poem for birthing

woman's life is not static. It changes with every moon, every season, and those changes are profound. Often women who begin their journey on a spiritual path become frustrated, even guilty, about their seeming inability to stick to a rigid program. It is not innate inability, but the inflexibility of male-oriented discipline that can cause these feelings, and can often cause women to abandon their spiritual practices altogether.

Psychologist Georgia Witkin Lanoil, in her book *The Female Stress Syndrome*, says that because girls are more often raised to be "good," that is, they are rewarded most when they conform and are considerate, women end up with an adulthood of impossible struggles. We try to be the perfect wife, mother, employee, and friend, often to our own detriment. When we adopt a spiritual path, we often try to be the perfect spiritual person. Unfortunately, the definition of perfection often excludes the natural phenomena of our lives.

The stresses that women experience are different from those of men. Women must cope with radical bodily changes — menstruation, pregnancy, childbirth, menopause. Psychological stresses arise from society's double messages: a homemaker feels pressured to have a career; a working mother feels pressured to spend more time with her children; a single woman is pressured to marry; the childless are pressured by time running out; the young mother worries about missing work and falling behind.

Women are often responsible for entertaining, chauffeuring, and their children's school and recreational activities in addition to housework, career, and marriage. Life changes such as marriage, divorce, and childbearing impact women much more profoundly because of the choices these changes force upon them. And women, every day, are subjected to the subtle but pervading stresses of unequal pay, double-duty work, sexual harassment, and sexism, all of which deplete, deny, and distract us.

Statistics bear this out. The death rate for women has stayed the same since 1950, while that for men has dropped. Though there has been a radical improvement in health care in the last thirty years, mortality for women has risen in proportion to it. The incidence of cancer and heart disease has risen for women as they have entered the workforce and faced the exhaustion and frustration of trying to "do it all."

External and internal stresses aggravate the natural stresses of bodily changes. For example, additional stresses such as deadlines or a sick child to care for just before menstruation can intensify premenstrual symptoms like acne or headaches. Stress affects the glandular secretions, which in turn cause many of these symptoms. Postpartum depression is very common and is often due to the combined impact of rapid hormonal shifts, changing roles and expectations, new financial worries, loss of freedom and choices, and lack of sleep. Menopause is another phase when women can be vulnerable to stress.

Again, on top of other pressures, shifts in brain chemistry can cause anxiety and depression. Women are more often socially stigmatized by aging, and since we live longer and earn less than men, the financial pressures increase as well.

Our society has created a difficult life for women, a situation that we, being over half the population, have the power to change. The stresses in our lives can be transformed by changing our perceptions and by finding new ways of relating to the world. Meditation, yoga, and other practices can help us balance our lives, eliminate unnecessary stress, and mentally reframe those sources of stress so that we can use them for our development. Spirituality can give us a strong center from which to work to change the pressures and prejudices that now work against us.

Your body changes with the cycles of the moon; so should your practices. Menstruation, pregnancy, nursing babies, raising small children, menopause: all these times change you not only physically but mentally and spiritually as well. Every woman will have her own way of growing through these changes, and I firmly believe in a flexible, intuitive approach. Here are some guidelines for the woman on the path of Tantra, as well as some philosophical points of view from women who have "been there," women whose years of spiritual discipline have been challenged by family life.

## MONTHLY CYCLES

If you don't chart your monthly cycles on a calendar, start now. Observe the effect that a shifting hormonal balance has on your energy, your vitality, your emotions, and your meditation. Many women experience a "heaviness" in their meditation a few days before menstruation begins, even if they perceive no other changes. Notice if your attitude toward meditation shifts during your period; are you more inclined toward it, or less? Knowing your natural inclinations can help you design your spiritual practices in a way that will assist rather than oppose you during this time.

Yoga postures should not be done during your period, a time when the delicate hormonal balance in your body shouldn't be disturbed. If you have menstrual difficulties, such as irregular cycles, heavy bleeding, cramping, or PMS, they can be addressed through yoga postures done regularly throughout the rest of the month. The postures and warm-ups in this book are very good for balancing women's hormones and strengthening the lower back and pelvic floor.

Kaoshikii can be done throughout the month and is very helpful as an energizing exercise before and during your period. Native healers have often spoken of menstruation as a woman's "time of power." As you become more attuned to the divine within, you will find this to be true. Kaoshikii strengthens the physical body, centers the mind, and channels the tremendous spiritual force coming through you at this time. Don't believe a culture that says you are weak and crazy once a month! Just the opposite is true. Your period can be a time of expanded awareness, when intuitive realization comes more easily. It is a good time to focus greater attention on your meditation. If because of physical discomfort you find meditation difficult, use the time for other things that will help nurture your spirit in solitude: reading, writing, walking in the woods or by the beach.

## PREGNANCY

Pregnancy can be one of the most spiritually alive times in your life; after all, a little person unfolding inside your body is living proof of the miracle of the universe. It is also a time when you'll get the most advice about the intimate details of your life from total strangers. I will leave all that to other people, and to the hundreds of other books on the subject, and confine myself to the "how to" (or not to, as the case may be) do your spiritual practices during this time, and how to keep your inner life growing amid the radical changes a new child brings.

**First Trimester:** In the first three months of your pregnancy, you may find yourself falling asleep at odd times, emotionally on edge, nauseated at different times of the day, and/or otherwise physically uneasy. Often women experience the same kind of difficulties they have had just before menstruation. All of your spiritual practices can continue during this time, but you may want to alter your schedule a bit, to allow yourself to sleep later in the morning and go to bed earlier at night. During my pregnancies, I became so tired by evening that I found it easier to do my first meditation in the morning and the second one at noon.

This is a time to be especially mindful of your diet and to get plenty of fresh air and exercise. Increase your protein intake from combinations of beans, legumes, grains, nuts, seeds, and dairy products. Boost your vitamins with fresh fruits, vegetables, and their juices.

**Second Trimester:** In the second few months, many of the physical discomforts of the early days disappear. You'll begin to feel the baby move; often a sense of well-being and positivity characterize this trimester. Yoga postures should stop, again because of the drastic hormonal shifts taking place and to avoid putting unnatural pressure upon the womb. Gentle stretching exercises can help ease discomforts and keep your body feeling good; Sandra Jordan's *Yoga for Pregnancy* is a good resource for these. You can continue practicing kaoshikii. This is the time to shore up your spirit with a lot of meditation. The baby needs spiritual energy, and you do, too, in preparation for the big job of parenting, when time for quiet meditation is hard to find.

It's time to begin communicating with your baby, and what better way than through your meditation? Set aside a certain time every day for your special meditation. Sit somewhere comfortable, close your eyes, and relax deeply. Place your hands on your belly and relax them. Feel your hands getting warm. Visualize your baby, and imagine the connection between you to be like a beautiful, golden figure-eight of light. Feel the love moving back and forth between you, getting stronger and stronger.

Talk to your baby. Say whatever comes to mind, and wait for a response; after awhile, you'll start to feel your baby responding to you. It may be just a sense, or it may appear in your mind as a voice or a picture, or you may feel baby move in a way that indicates response. Have no doubt that this communication is real, that you have the spiritual power to deeply connect with your baby, even at this early stage.

What does your baby need? Imagine yourself in that little body, growing inside the womb; what do you need? When you feel the link between you and your baby, you can even ask him or her, "What do you need? What can I do for you?" and get an answer. You may want to write down your experiences from these meditations; you may perceive messages that you don't understand at the moment, but will later upon looking back.

**Third Trimester:** In the last few months physical discomfort may return as the baby uses more of your energy for that last growth spurt, and as his or her weight imposes more on your resources. Your special meditations will become very strong these last few months; already you have established a strong bond of communication and respect that will help you understand your baby after he or she is born.

When you sit for your regular meditation, you may want some added support; an extra pillow underneath or the support of leaning against a wall should help ease the discomfort of sitting. Kaoshikii, though a bit cumbersome, is one of the best childbirth preparation exercises. It strengthens and stretches all the supportive muscles around the pelvis and back and helps open up the pelvic floor. In addition, you'll want to do extra back-strengthening exercises and squatting movements to help loosen any tightness in the pelvic area.

Schedule yourself for a full body massage several times during this last trimester. Not only will it help you relax, but studies have shown that a mother who is touched and massaged regularly during her pregnancy is more confident handling her baby later on. Massage your belly every day with a light, natural oil such as almond or avocado oil. Feel your hands massage your baby, sending loving, relaxing energy to him or her.

Pay attention to your dreams and intuitive insights during this period. Write everything down. Surround yourself with beauty in color, nature, music. Read inspiring books, and sing. The preparation of your spirit for the coming of your child is at least as important as physical and mental preparation, if not more.

## BIRTH

Because the birth of your baby will be attended by such an overwhelming amount of advice, I will refrain from adding to it, except to say that it is important, of course, to prepare for it physically, mentally, and spiritually, to try to plan the most gentle and loving welcome possible. At the same time, surrender to whatever your samskaras may bring, and be willing to make beautiful whatever circumstances unfold at the final hour. The birth is important, but more significant are the next twenty years (and beyond) of your relationship with this new companion on your path.

## A NEWBORN IN THE HOUSE

A Native American story: There was once a great chief who had done everything, who had seen everything, and who was very, very proud.

He walked through the village saying, "I am the greatest chief there is."

An old woman came up to the chief and said, "No you're not. I know a greater chief than you."

"What do you mean?" thundered the chief. "There is no chief greater than me."

The old woman challenged him. "If you come to my hogan tomorrow at noon," she said, "I will introduce you to this great chief."

"Very well, Grandmother," said the chief. "I will be there tomorrow at noon."

The chief went home and slept very soundly in order to gain strength and beauty during the night. In the morning he put on his finest clothing, his eagle headdress, his medicine beads, and his buckskin leggings.

When he was finished he knew that if it were a contest of strength or beauty, he would win.

He went to the woman's house and said, "Grandmother! I am here. It is noon." He went inside and saw the old woman, and a baby crawling around on the floor.

He looked around and said, "Where is the great chief you spoke of?"

"You see him in front of you, Oh Chief," said the woman.

"What do you mean?" the chief blustered. "This is a baby. Are you trying to play a trick on me?"

The baby was frightened by the sudden, angry loud voice and started to cry. The chief became very flustered and pulled off his eagle headdress and brushed the baby's cheeks with the feathers. He pulled off his medicine beads and dangled them in front of the baby's nose; he pulled off all of his baubles and bangles and jingled them in the baby's ears.

At last the baby stopped crying, and the grandmother said, "See? The baby won the battle. Even you, the great chief, had to stop talking to care for the baby. In every hogan, the baby is the greatest chief, for everyone loves and obeys the baby implicitly."

"You are right, Grandmother," the chief replied. "You and the baby chief have taught me a great lesson." He put on his beads and feathers and turned to go, and as he did, the baby called out, "Goo!"

So ever since then, babies all over the world say "Goo." It means, "I am the greatest chief!"

For the first year of his or her life, your baby is "chief." This is a special time, and it passes quickly, never to return. More than anything, your baby needs your physical proximity — to hear your voice, to feel your touch, to be welcomed, reassured, and loved.

Often parents will find that the baby wakes up or starts to fuss when they begin to meditate. Perhaps the baby senses your withdrawal and feels afraid or lonely. There are several remedies — you'll have to experiment to find what works for you. Some parents are so taxed by the baby's demands and household work those first months that they cannot sit down for regular meditation. Others find that meditation helps keep them centered and increases their stamina, so they make it a priority. If possible, have a partner look after the baby while you do your meditation, at least once a day.

You can continue your special meditations. While nursing or massaging your baby, imagine the energy of love between you, feel your connection to the whole universe. In this way, your baby won't feel shut out by your spiritual practices, but will be a part of them.

Sometimes parents who are overly attached to their disciplines will inadvertently establish an adversarial relationship with their babies by insisting upon keeping rigid schedules regardless of the baby's needs. This is unfortunate, because often our children are much more spiritually evolved than we are; if we include them and respect them, we can learn from them. If not, we risk alienating them and miss the point of our spiritual effort altogether.

You can resume yoga postures, if all is well, when your baby is around four to five months old.

## LIFE WITH YOUNG CHILDREN

Many women experience drastic changes in their spiritual lives with the birth of their children. Some say that withdrawal of the mind in meditation becomes painful or impossible, with a mother's eyes, ears, and heart so attuned to her children. This is especially true with children under five or six years of age; it does change as they grow older. You may need to alter your expectations during this period. Each phase of life brings a different kind of growth, and demands a different kind of practice. The early years of parenthood require the practice of "living meditation" more than other times in your life, when you might place those same energies into your sitting meditations. Each phase, if approached with a sincere desire to grow, will offer the precise tools you need at the moment.

During the hectic years of early parenthood you may long for the tranquility of peaceful meditation without the bonds of love and responsibility that seem to tie you to the earth. But this earth, too, requires mastery; those loving responsibilities, too, move you toward the goal. When you long for the world beyond and worry that you may have lost your spiritual discipline, take a moment to look at your life in a broader context. What are you learning right now? How is your life teaching you spiritual lessons that you will use later? You will probably discover that these earthly "bondages" are some of your most powerful teachers. When you are able to sit for meditation again, you will find a one-pointed concentration has developed during those years of "scattered" energies. A deeper ideation is possible because of the work you have done at the level of the heart. You are able to truly give yourself to your spiritual quest because you have learned how to give.

## SEXUALITY

The word *Tantra* means "liberation through mental expansion" or "liberation from crudeness and stagnation," depending upon how the syllables are translated. The basic tenet of Tantric philosophy is that absolute reality is neutral, having two aspects: pure consciousness (Shiva) and the operative principle (Shakti). This universe is the result of the union of Shiva and Shakti; manifestation occurs as Shakti binds Shiva into different forms. Ancient teachers described this subtle concept in terms that people could understand: the symbol of man and woman joining in sexual communion. People could relate to the profundity of "two-in-one" through their own experience.

Tantra originated in matriarchal times in India, when women were teachers who passed secret knowledge down through generations. Shakti was "Mother," the supreme cognitive force, and Shiva was the operative principle. The goal of spiritual practice was, as it is today, to merge in that pure blissful consciousness. Sexuality was a natural symbol of that merger.

With the invasion of the patriarchal, warlike Aryan tribes, things began to change. The caste system developed, whereby lighter-skinned people placed themselves above the darker-skinned natives who worshipped the Mother Goddess and had originated Tantric traditions. The interpretation of symbols began to change; eventually Shakti (seen as feminine) was the operative principle, subordinate to Shiva (seen as masculine). The idea was to throw off the shackles of nature (Shakti) in order to merge in Shiva. A split between nature and spirit emerged, and women symbolized the "demoness" nature that held consciousness (men) in bondage.

In ancient religions sexuality was very much a part of life, not hidden or unclean, and could be a means to spiritual development. This changed with the advent of patriarchal domination, and women, whose bodies symbolized the power of nature and sexuality, were seen as enemies of spiritual enlightenment, to be subjugated and controlled by the men who had usurped their spiritual power.

Though the ancient symbols still live in thousands of confusing forms, interpretations, and dogmas, modern Tantrics are reaching beyond the masculine/feminine symbology to a holistic, humanistic view of creation and the spiritual journey. Woman are reclaiming their place on the spiritual path and bringing feminine power back into the picture. A balanced, progressive outlook and philosophy is now beginning to reemerge. When nature is no longer perceived as the enemy to be conquered, and light-skinned males are no longer the accepted rulers of religion and society, a radical shift will have taken place that allows the growth and development of humanity in cooperation with all the other creatures on our planet.

There are several different schools of Tantra, and many practical approaches as well. One form of Tantric practice, called The Five Ms is the basis for the so-called Tantra of Sex that you may have heard or read about. The Five Ms are a portion of ancient Tantric ritual that had both physical and spiritual meanings. Some scholars say the literal version was meant as a stepping-stone for those who were unable to do a more subtle form of practice — those whose animal instincts were still quite strong. It was meant to spiritualize the things of everyday life. Thus, the activities of everyday life such as sexuality could come to be an expression of spirituality and worship.

## THE FIVE MS
   (1) *Mamsa Sadhana.* Literal meaning: ritual consumption of meat. Subtle meaning: to control the tongue (speech).
   (2) *Matsya Sadhana.* Literal meaning: ritual consumption of fish. Subtle

meaning: to control the respiration (pranayama).

(3) *Madya Sadhana*. Literal meaning: ritual consumption of wine. Subtle meaning: to control the nectar that, it is said, is secreted by the pineal gland when the body becomes very subtle, and that creates an ecstatic feeling.

(4) *Mudra Sadhana*. Literal meaning: the use of symbols in ritual. Subtle meaning: to control the propensities (vrttis) through spiritual practices such as yoga postures.

(5) *Maethun Sadhana*. Literal meaning: ritual sexual intercourse. Subtle meaning: the mystic union of Shiva and Shakti through deep meditation.

There is debate as to whether the literal translations of these practices were actually religious doctrine or, more likely, codes that referred to the subtle practices. Much of Tantra has been passed down in code through thousands of years from teacher to student. Tantra provided, and still provides, a context in which all of life is spiritualized. Tantra is not the "yoga of sex," it is the yoga of everything. Tantra does not favor suppression of the instincts, but rather control, whereby the mind is always directed toward spirituality. Freud spoke of the libido (sexual energy) as a force that doesn't necessarily have a sexual goal; in this, he was in agreement with Tantric teachings. This powerful energy, which may be expressed in sexual intercourse, can also be used for spiritual attainment.

Casual sex can be harmful physically, emotionally, and spiritually, just as drugs, liquor, or food are in excess. Used with addiction like an intoxicant, sex becomes destructive, drawing off vital energy that can be used in creative and spiritual pursuits. Sexuality can be a much deeper expression than this. Between two lovers who care deeply for one another and whose spiritual and emotional sensitivity is mature, sexual communication can reinforce spiritual goals and commitment. It is then a sacred enactment of the essential spiritual drama — the bliss of universal oneness.

## LATER LIFE

The saying "life begins at forty" has never been so true for women as it is today. The myth that menopause is a negative experience is dispelled as women claim their personal power. A new life can open up as children grow and we find more time to direct our inner and outer lives toward our own goals. As Margaret Mead once said, "The most creative force in the world is the menopausal woman with zest." Later life can be a time when a new spiritual awareness grows. Experience and wisdom augment new possibilities; a greater self-assurance allows us to place priority on our self-development.

For many of us, menopause is a challenging adjustment, when the body's wisdom must be honored — or else! It is time to love and validate your body more than you ever have, and that means to learn what it needs to be happy. Use your yoga session as a time of rest and rejuvenation. Put on music that makes you smile, slow down, and consciously send love and acceptance to every area of your body. If your mind resists or wants to jump in with negative thoughts, pessimistic scenarios, and fears, send a wave of loving kindness to that fearful part of yourself each time you breathe in or out.

Physical and emotional discomforts that may be experienced during menopause can be greatly alleviated by good nutrition, yoga, exercise, and meditation. Many health professionals now recommend these natural

As we become more mechanized and urbanized, our contact with the Earth and nature becomes more frail, and with it our health and sense of self-worth. Our power is transferred to the upper body where it is tenuous and must be constantly guarded.

When too much abrasive energy is found in our surroundings, the chakras will close down to protect the subtle body from this caustic invasion.

—— Anodea Judith,
*Wheels of Life*

techniques and supplements to augment — even replace — estrogen therapy. If you do take estrogen, you might consider consulting your doctor about reducing the dosage once you are established in daily yoga, exercise, and a healthy vegetarian or semivegetarian diet supplemented with calcium and vitamins. You may wish to explore herbal or homeopathic remedies.

Read up on this important passage in your life, much as you may have read books on pregnancy and childbirth. What an exciting time! No longer do women face the "empty nest" and a rocking chair as later life approaches. Rather, with the strength and inner beauty afforded by regular meditation practice, we can begin a new phase of growth and fulfillment.

This is the promise of Tantra Yoga: Every phase of life we pass through is a new phase of physical, emotional, mental, and spiritual growth and fulfillment.

---

Recommended Reading:

*Yoga for Pregnancy: 92 Safe and Gentle Stretches* by Sandra Jordan

*Essential Exercises for the Childbearing Year* by Elizabeth Noble

*Infant Massage, a Handbook for Loving Parents* by Vimala McClure

*Whole Child Whole Parent* by Polly Berrien Berends

*Menopause Naturally: Preparing for the Second Half of Life* by Sadja Greenwood, M.D.

# Glossary

**Ahimsa:** the first principle of the Tantric Code of Ethics: simple kindness. Literal meaning is "nonharm."

**Ajina Chakra:** the sixth chakra; literal meaning is "perception plexus."

**Anahata Chakra:** the fourth chakra; literal meaning is "pure plexus."

**Annamaya Kosa:** the first layer of the mind (which is the body); literal meaning is "made of food."

**Aparigraha:** the fifth principle of the Tantric Code of Ethics: simplicity. Literal meaning is "nonacquisition."

**Asana(s):** physical exercises that harmonize the glandular system and thus can make the body fit for meditation.

**Asteya:** the third principle of the Tantric Code of Ethics: responsibility. Literal meaning is "nontheft."

**Atimanasa Kosa:** the supramental layer of mind; literal meaning is "higher mind."

**Aunkara (Aum):** the sound of creation; sometimes heard in deep meditation. "A" is the creation, "U" is the maintenance of balance, "M(a)" is the destructive force.

**Astaunga Yoga:** an eightfold system of yoga practice organized by the sage Patanjali in India, based on earlier work by the yoga master Astavarka. Literal meaning of astaunga is "eight parts."

**Babanam Kevalam:** a universal mantra used in chanting and meditation, meaning "all is one." (Babanam means "the name of the Creator"; Kevalam means "is all there is.")

**Brahma:** the infinite consciousness from which everything arises.

**Brahmachakra:** the cycle of creation; the movement of consciousness from its infinite state into matter and then from the dense to the subtle, merging again in pure consciousness.

**Brahmacharya:** the fourth principle of the Tantric Code of Ethics: perceiving everything as an expression of the Creator. Literal meaning is "to follow God."

**Chakra(s):** nuclei located throughout the body's subtle structure; foci of psychic energy.

223

**Dharma**: "innate tendency," that which propels every living being toward oneness with the Creator.

**Guru**: "that which dispels darkness," according to Tantra, the only true Guru is infinite consciousness.

**Guru Puja**: the practice of surrendering all our fears and desires to the higher self after meditation.

**Hiranyamaya Kosa**: the subtle causal or "superconscious" layer of mind; literal meaning is "golden."

**Iishvara Pranidhana**: the tenth principle of the Tantric Code of Ethics: spirituality. Literal meaning is "taking shelter in the Supreme Being."

**Iccha Shakti:** spiritual force developed by meditation and right conduct.

**Kama**: limited desires.

**Kamamaya Kosa**: the conscious layer of mind; literal meaning is "desire."

**Karma:** the result of samskaras; the reaction experienced as a result of actions and desires.

**Kaoshikii**: a dancing exercise that vitalizes the body, focuses the mind, and strengthens the will.

**Kosa(s)**: the layers of the mind.

**Kundalini**: spiritual energy residing in every living being.

**Manipura Chakra:** the third chakra; literal meaning is "fiery plexus."

**Manomaya Kosa**: the subconscious layer of mind; literal meaning is "mental."

**Mantra**: a collection of sound vibrations used as a focus in meditation.

**Muladhara Chakra:** the first chakra; literal meaning is "root plexus."

**Nadii(s)**: psychic pathways that channel energy through the chakras.

**Niyama:** five healthy practices that compose half of the Tantric Code of Ethics.

**Prana**: vital energy.

**Pranayama**: control of the vital energy through the practice of meditation with breathing exercises.

**Pranendriya**: the "sixth sense;" actually a type of psychic organ that regulates mental and physical functions.

**Prema**: limitless love.

**Rajadhiraja Yoga**: the first known teachings of yoga master Astavarka in India, 2,000 years ago. Literal meaning of rajadhiraja: is "king of kings."

**Rjuta**: straightforwardness in character; a quality developed through proper meditation and right conduct.

**Rta**: the absolute truth, with or without the spirit of kindness.

**Sadhana:** meditation; literal meaning is "the effort that brings enlightenment."

**Sahasrara Chakra:** the seventh chakra; literal meaning is "thousand-petaled lotus plexus."

**Samadhi:** a state achieved in meditation, wherein one experiences oneness with the Creator.

**Samskara(s):** inborn, acquired, or imposed reactive momenta from past thoughts and actions, stored in the mind and expressed as "fate."

**Santosa:** the seventh principle of the Tantric Code of Ethics: acceptance. Literal meaning is "with contentment."

**Satya:** the second principle of the Tantric Code of Ethics: honesty. Literal meaning is "truth with the spirit of kindness."

**Shakti:** "operative principle;" that which binds infinite consciousness to finite form.

**Shaoca:** the sixth principle of the Tantric Code of Ethics: clarity. Literal meaning is "clean."

**Shiva:** infinite consciousness, unbound; also, the name of a great Tantric Guru who lived in ancient India.

**Susumna:** the "psychic canal" through which the kundalini energy is channeled.

**Svadhisthana Chakra:** the second chakra; literal meaning is "sweet plexus."

**Svadhyaya:** the ninth principle of the Tantric Code of Ethics: understanding. Literal meaning is "study of Self."

**Tantra:** the ancient spiritual discipline upon which yoga is based.

**Tapah:** the eighth principle of the Tantric Code of Ethics: service. Literal meaning is "penance or sacrifice."

**Vijinanamaya Kosa:** the subliminal layer of mind; literal meaning is "special knowledge."

**Vishuddha Chakra:** the fifth chakra; literal meaning is "purification plexus."

**Vrtti(s):** psychic propensities, such as lust, hope, etc., located within and controlled by the chakras.

**Yama:** five acts of integrity that compose half of the Tantric Code of Ethics.

**Yoga:** "union" of the self with infinite consciousness; the practices that bring that union, including the eight parts of Austaunga Yoga as given by the sage Patanjali.

**Yogi:** practitioner of yoga.

# About the Author

Vimala McClure is a writer and award-winning textile artist living in Boulder, Colorado. Her books include *Infant Massage: A Handbook for Loving Parents* (Bantam), *The Tao of Motherhood* (New World Library), and *Bangladesh* (Simon & Schuster). Vimala has been practicing Tantra Yoga since 1971.

# For Information and Instruction

The Progressive Women's Spiritual Association offers classes and personal instruction in meditation, yoga, vegetarian diet, and spiritual philosophy. For further information, write to: PWSA, 97-38 42nd Ave., Corona, NY 11368-2145.

# Suggested Reading

*Beyond the Superconscious Mind*
by Avtk. Ananda Mitra Ac.

*Einstein's Space and Van Gogh's Sky: Physical Reality and Beyond* by Lawrence LeShan and Henry Margeneau

*Essential Exercises for the Childbearing Year* by Elizabeth Noble

*Everyday Ethics* by Joshua Halberstam

*A Guide to Human Conduct* by P.R. Sarkar

*Infant Massage: A Handbook for Loving Parents* by Vimala McClure

*Menopause Naturally: Preparing for the Second Half of Life* by Sadja Greenwood, M.D.

*Reincarnation: a New Horizon in Science, Religion, and Society* by Sylvia Cranston and Carey Williams

*The Relaxation and Stress Reduction Workbook* by Martha Davis, Matthew McKay, and Beth Eshelman

*The Tao of Physics* by Fritjof Capra

*Up from Eden* by Ken Wilbur

*The Vegetarian Alternative* edited by Vimala McClure

*Vegetarian Food for All* by Annabel Perkins

*The Vegetarian Lunchbasket* by Linda Haynes

*Whole Child, Whole Parent* by Polly Berrien Berends

*Woman Spirit: A Guide to Women's Wisdom* by Hallie Iglehart

*A Woman's Book of Confidence* by Sue Patton Thoele

*A Woman's Book of Spirit* by Sue Patton Thoele

*Yoga for Pregnancy: 92 Safe and Gentle Stretches* by Sandra Jordan

New World Library is dedicated to
publishing books and cassettes that inspire
and challenge us to improve the quality
of our lives and our world.

Our books and tapes are available
in bookstores everywhere.
For a catalog of our complete library
of fine books and cassettes, contact:

New World Library
14 Pamaron Way
Novato, CA 94949
Phone: (415) 884-2100
Fax: (415) 884-2199
Or call toll-free: (800) 972-6657
Catalog Requests: Ext. 900
Ordering: Ext. 902
Email: escort@nwlib.com